YOGA FOR BEGINNERS: HATHA YOGA

The Complete Guide to Master Hatha Yoga; Benefits, Essentials, Asanas (with Pictures), Precautions, Common Mistakes, FAQs, and Common Myths

Rohit Sahu

Published by: Rohit Sahu
Contact: rohit@rohitsahu.net
Published Worldwide

➤ I highly acknowledge Yogi Gorakhnath for his contribution to Hatha Yoga. He is called the founder of Hatha yoga, together with his master Matsyendranath, although many of the tenets and practices of this school were in existence long before his time.

➤ Yogi Gorakhnath (also known as Goraksanath, c. early 11th century) was a Hindu yogi, saint and one of the earliest poets of Bhojpuri, who was the influential founder of the Nath Hindu monastic movement in India. He is considered as one of the two notable disciples of Matsyendranath.

➤ I highly acknowledge all the people whose pictures I've used in this book to illustrate poses.

CONTENTS

AUTHOR NOTE

Dear Reader,

With great excitement and appreciation, I offer to you this book, the culmination of my Ayurvedic and spiritual studies. It's been a labor of love, knitted together to impart timeless knowledge and practical insights to improve your knowledge on the subject of Yoga. I urge you to go on a transforming journey as you read through the pages of this book. Explore various Asanas (poses), Pranayamas (breathwork), and deep knowledge that you may incorporate into your everyday life.

Your thoughts and opinions are really valuable to me. I would be grateful if you could take a few seconds to leave a review on Amazon and share your ideas and experiences. Your review will not only help other readers make an informed decision, but it will also give vital insight into how this book has touched your life.

I sincerely ask you to share your thoughts, observations, and any recommendations you may have. Your thoughts will not only encourage me but will also help to evolve and refine the information and wisdom contained inside these pages.

May this book serve as a beacon of light for you on your journey to self-discovery, health, and spiritual advancement. Thank you for joining me on this journey.

With the deepest gratitude,

Rohit Sahu

INTRODUCTION

Yoga's origin can be traced back to more than 5,000 years ago, but some researchers believe that yoga may be up to 10,000 years old. The word 'Yoga' first appeared in the oldest sacred texts, the Rig Veda, and is derived from the Sanskrit root "Yuj" which means to unite.

Yoga is primarily a spiritual discipline that focuses on subtle science, on achieving harmony between the mind and the body of the individual. According to the yoga scriptures, the practice of yoga leads an individual to a union of consciousness with that of universal consciousness. It eventually leads to a great harmony between the human mind and body, man and nature.

The Vedas is a series of texts comprising songs, mantras, and practices used by the Vedic priests, the Brahmans. Yoga was slowly refined and developed by the Brahman and Rishis (mystical seers) who documented their practice and belief in the Upanishads, a vast work containing more than 200 scriptures.

According to modern philosophers, anything in the world is merely a reflection of the same quantum firmament. One who experiences this oneness of life is considered being in yoga and is referred to as 'Yogi,' having achieved a condition of liberation referred to as Mukti, Nirvana, or Moksha. So the goal of yoga is self-realization, to overcome all kinds of sufferings leading to 'The State of Liberation' (Moksha) or 'Freedom' (Kaivalya).

And yoga is not just for spiritual progress, it provides multiple health advantages as well, such as enhancing endurance, reducing depression, and improving overall wellness and fitness. It's a wonderful mind-body practice that encourages relaxation when you practice linking breathwork (Pranayama) to poses (Asanas). In addition, a recent study has also related the benefits of all types of yoga to enhanced bone density and better sleep quality.

As yoga has grown into mainstream popularity, many styles and variations have emerged in the wellness space. This centuries-old Eastern philosophy is now widely practiced and taught by people of all ages, sizes, and backgrounds.

There are 10 primary types of yoga. With so many different types, it may be a little difficult to determine which type is appropriate for you. But remember that there's no right or wrong—just that one might not be right for you at this moment.

You've to ask yourself what's important to you in your yoga practice: Are you searching for a sweaty, intense practice? Or are you searching for a more meditative, gentler practice that looks more appealing?

Like any sort of exercise, choose something you want to do; Bikram or Iyengar will attract you if you're a detailed person. If you're more of a free spirit, Vinyasa or Aerial yoga could be fun.

I've made a complete series on all 10 types of yoga. This is Hatha Yoga; others are also available!

So, What is Hatha Yoga?

Hatha is a general category that includes most styles of yoga. It is an old system that includes the practice of Asanas and Pranayamas, which help bring peace to mind and body and prepares the body for deeper spiritual practices such as meditation. It emphasizes the cultivation of the body as a way of attaining a state of spiritual purity in which the mind is removed from external objects.

In India, Hatha Yoga in popular tradition is associated with the Yogis of Natha Sampradaya through its traditional founder,

Matsyendranath. Almost all Hathayogic texts belong to the Nath Siddhas, and the important ones are attributed to the disciples of Matsyendranath, Gorakhnath, or Gorakshanath.

Hatha Yoga, once considered to be the mother of all other forms, is now seen in the West as their sibling. All the forms of yoga that you know—Iyengar, Ashtanga, Vinyasa, Kundalini, Power, Sivananda, Yin, Viniyoga, Restorative, Moksha, Kripalu, Forrest, Jivamukti, Anusara, and Bikram—come from what was once a full-life path and moral code called Hatha Yoga. But in today's world, Hatha Yoga is just another form of yoga.

Hatha Yoga is a preparatory process of yoga. The word "Ha" means the sun, and "Ta" means the moon. "Hatha" means a yoga that brings the equilibrium between the sun and the moon within you, or Pingala and Ida within you. You can pursue Hatha Yoga in ways that carry you beyond certain limits, but essentially, it's a physical preparation—preparing the body for a higher possibility.

Hatha Yoga has become a popular form of exercise in many parts of the world. It's easy accessibility and emphasis on health and well-being has made it play an important role in counteracting the many harmful impacts of a rapidly changing world.

Hatha Yoga has grown in popularity as an exercise that improves strength, endurance, relaxation, and focus of mind. It offers an opportunity to stretch, unwind, and reduce stress, offering a strong counterpoint to both busy lives and aerobic exercises. As with any other yoga practice, it can be done by anyone, regardless of sexuality, race, class, or creed.

Training involves breath, body, and mind, and sessions typically require 45-90 minutes of breathing, yoga poses, and meditation.

Today, the word Hatha is used in such a vague context that it is impossible to realize what a specific Hatha Yoga session is going to be like. In most cases, though, it will be relatively gentle, slow, and perfect for beginners or students who want a more relaxed approach where yoga poses are kept longer.

This Hatha Yoga guide is perfect for beginners and those looking for a more mindful practice. It will strengthen and stretch the body, keeping each pose for several breaths. If you're new to yoga, recovering from injury, or looking to relax by moving gently and thoughtfully, this yoga style might be the best fit for you.

All you've got to do is show up. When you decide to take care of yourself, all kinds of good things begin to happen. You'll have more energy. You'll become relaxed. Your attitude to life will turn more optimistic. And all of these changes you'll undergo on this yoga journey will continue to affect those around you in ways you've never dreamed of.

This practice will offer optimistic, loving energy that will spread across the universe. And as you deepen your yoga practice, you will have the chance to meet a lot of like-minded souls like yourself.

Hatha Yoga has countless benefits. The slower flow—relative to Vinyasa or Power Yoga—can feel less challenging and encourage the practitioner to develop comfort with the poses.

It's perfect for those looking for a gentle, basic yoga routine. It's the ideal practice to calm down and relax, but it's also the best practice to keep the body active!

In this session, you will have the freedom to work on your alignment, practice relaxing techniques, and feel comfortable practicing yoga while developing strength and endurance.

Hatha Yoga rituals—including Asanas, Pranayamas, Mudras, Mantras, and Meditation—cultivate strong energies to promote improvement both mentally and physically. They will change the way you feel in your soul and body.

Not only can Hatha Yoga boost positive emotions and well-being, but it can also relieve depression and sorrow as well as promote relaxation. Overall, we can use this yoga practice to feel more connected to ourselves and to the world we live in.

Hatha Yoga poses and breathing exercises are believed to purify the physical body. Even if you've formed any bad habits, by doing Hatha Yoga, you'll lose all unnecessary cravings. Hatha Yoga and its adaptations have also been found to enhance immunity, minimize symptoms of aging, control hormones, and facilitate healthy blood flow.

So, are you interested in learning all about how Hatha Yoga can benefit you? This is a comprehensive guide to take a closer look at what this gentle and slow-paced yoga style can do for you and how you can master it for your overall well-being.

Covering the fundamentals of each practice in-depth and how to correct the most common errors, this Hatha Yoga Guide has left nothing to help you attain mental, spiritual, and physical well-being.

SCIENCE BEHIND HATHA YOGA

Hatha Yoga benefits from a comprehensive understanding of the body's mechanics and uses yogic postures to allow the body to retain higher energy dimensions. By pursuing this profound science, you will improve and strengthen the way you perceive, behave, and experience life. Hatha Yoga is about building a body that isn't a hindrance to your life. The body becomes a stepping stone in the progression toward the blooming of the ultimate possibility.

Hatha Yoga is not an exercise, it's a science! Why? First, it's based on the universal aspects of human behavior. Second, it relies on actual knowledge, not on assumptions. Third, anyone doing Hatha Yoga would reap the expected benefits.

Understanding the complexities of the body, building a certain aura, and then utilizing body poses to direct energy in a specific way is what Hatha Yoga is all about.

Hatha Yoga relates to the balancing of the masculine aspects (active, hot, sun) with feminine aspects (receptive, cool, moon) within all of us. Hatha Yoga is a road to harmony and to merging opposites. We establish a combination of strength and flexibility in our physical bodies. We also learn to align our energies and surrender in each pose.

Hatha Yoga is an effective self-transforming technique. It encourages us to bring our focus to our breath, which allows us to keep up with the fluctuations of our minds and to be more involved in the unfolding of each moment.

In order to get the best out of Hatha Yoga practice, you need some inner resources and knowledge to function successfully on the subtle layers of your being. Practices in this book will help you develop these inner resources.

Today, the Hatha Yoga that people practice is not in its classical form, not in its maximum scope and dimension. Some of the 'Hatha Yoga Studios' that you see today just teach the physical side of it.

Hatha Yoga is not about bending your body, balancing on your head, or holding your breath. There was a time when people would explode with joy; tears of happiness would spill just doing asanas. That's the way yoga ought to be performed. Unfortunately, Hatha Yoga in the world today provides peace to some, is healthy to others, and is a painful circus to many.

Every day, you encounter part of the clear context of Hatha Yoga —your state of mind induces certain motions of energy within your body, and these motions, in essence, influence your bodily location. It's plain body language.

For example, disappointment, lethargy, and drowsiness allow energy to drain down, away from the brain. That flow, in turn, affects your posture—you appear to collapse, as though you shut yourself off from life. The very terms you use also show the downward movement: "I feel depressed," "I feel low," or "I feel sad."

On the other hand, pleasure, passion, and creativity allow energy to flood upward toward the brain, which then comes alive. You straighten up into a spacious, life-asserting stance. You inhale as if to welcome the world—and you're happy. Your words, too, convey the upward flow: "I feel at the top of the world," "I am happy," or "I feel optimistic."

You've definitely witnessed all this, even if you haven't seen it as a chain of influence—the mind influences energy, which in turn influences the body.

Each of the several asanas and pranayamas of Hatha Yoga has its specific influence on energy and consciousness. You can pair these practices with an overall routine that delivers plentiful, relaxed, concentrated energy to the brain. This will boost your consciousness, training you for the most important and powerful technique in yoga—Meditation.

When a person steps through deeper realms of meditation, it provides a greater likelihood of energy. If you want the energy to rise up, the body's pipeline (Nadis) must be favorable. If it's blocked, it won't function, or else something will burst. It is really important to train the body adequately until one enters into deeper meditation. Hatha Yoga ensures that your body takes it slowly and joyfully.

It implies that you want to make the comfort zone universal instead of the tiny band that's right now. Whoever and wherever you might be, you're at peace. You will naturally attain a composition of health, joy, bliss, and above all, balance. It's a very powerful way of living.

Finally, talking of the spiritual aspect, the correct combination of science and art, and of self-effort and grace, along with a living relationship with the soul, are key to a meaningful approach to Hatha Yoga. There is no hidden recipe for the right balance; it is highly personal. You will discover it in your own experiment—and, when you do, an entire universe of joy-filled opportunities will open up to you.

WHO CAN PERFORM IT?

1. Do you want to enhance mental tranquility, physical health, and divine influence?

2. Are you looking to strengthen your core muscles and strength?

3. Are you looking for a gentle, mindful yoga practice?

4. Do you want to get a better night's sleep?

5. Do you want to fill your life with strength, courage, flexibility, peace, opulence, balance, and perfection?

6. Are you looking to balance, harmonize, and unite the two fundamental energies in your system, your solar and lunar energies?

7. Do you want to improve depression symptoms?

8. Are you looking for a permanent solution to your stress?

9. Do you want to lose weight?

10. Do you wish to have stronger immunity?

11. Do you want healthy and glowing skin?

12. Do you want to improve your heart health?

13. Do you have weak bone density?

14. Is your lifestyle messed up and you want to develop discipline and self-control?

15. Are you looking for a way to prepare the body for meditation?

16. Do you want to enhance the quality of Prana?

17. Do you want to advance your spiritual growth?

18. Do you want to attain overall well-being?

If you replied "YES" to any of these issues, you should perform Hatha Yoga. It will offer an optimistic, loving energy that will spread across the universe. You will naturally attain a composition of health, joy, bliss, and above all, balance; an entire universe of joy-filled opportunities will open up to you.

BENEFITS OF HATHA YOGA

Hatha Yoga provides numerous advantages. Start your practice and witness some of the most notable ones.

1. Improves Cardiac Health

Daily performance of Hatha Yoga postures keeps the health risk of Hypertension in check—the major cause of heart disease. Hatha Yoga often decreases symptoms of anginal discomfort, increases blood supply to the heart, and heals the heart lesion for proper functioning. A study has found that it also enhances how blood travels to the heart, and the heart lesions are indicative of the disease.

Certain yoga poses boost cardiovascular health, enhance lung capacity, and enhance respiratory efficiency. They also encourage calmness and relief, reducing the incidence of hypertension, which is one of the major causes of cardiac disorders. They also boost blood supply and reduce inflammation.

Hatha Yoga poses often stretch muscles, rendering them more receptive to insulin, which is essential for blood sugar control. Then yoga poses require intense relaxation to ease blood pressure. Mind-calming meditation is another vital aspect of Hatha Yoga to relieve the nervous system and stress. All of these practices will help prevent disease.

Some of the best Hatha Yoga poses for the heart are Mountain Pose, Big Toe Pose, Bridge Pose, and Lion's Breath.

2. Enhances Your Overall Fitness

Hatha Yoga poses boost various facets of physical fitness when practiced regularly. As seen in a study reported in 2001, a minimum of two yoga lessons each week—including 10 minutes of active warm-up and 50 minutes of asana—for eight weeks' boosts oxygen absorption, muscle strength and agility, and joint mobility.

3. Helps Develop Discipline and Self-Control

A lot of importance is given to how Hatha Yoga impacts the well-being of the human body. But the practice is just as much of a mental one. While we're doing a yoga pose, we're getting the body out of its regular comfort zone and keeping a calm, equanimous state of mind.

This will help us build discipline and self-control in our everyday lives, resolve mild cravings and addictions, and also strengthen our relationships with others.

4. Boosts Bone Density

Yoga will improve your strength and agility, thus guarding you against falling, which is a major cause of osteoporotic fractures. Low bone density or osteopenia can trigger bone fractures or minimal trauma. It also causes thin and delicate bones that characterize the condition of osteoporosis.

Although having the right diet is necessary to make the bone healthier, Hatha Yoga is helpful in the treatment of bone loss as it facilitates bone density.

Weight-bearing yoga poses—such as Tree, Side Angle, Triangle, and Warrior I, II, and III reverse bone deterioration in people with osteoporosis and osteopenia. Research published in 2016 found that just 12 minutes of daily practice would enhance bone density in the spine and the femur.

In such poses, you use one group of muscles against another, such as the quad against the hamstrings or the gluteal muscles against the shoulder muscles. It produces an effect that actively triggers osteoblasts, which are bone-forming cells that are originally located outside the bone and transform into osteocytes. These cells are absorbed into the bone. This phenomenon will give rise to new bone.

5. Prepares the Body for Meditation

Hatha Yoga provides a lot of physical well-being advantages. However, it is necessary not to lose sight of the fact that yoga is a spiritual practice designed to draw the practitioner into increasingly deeper states of self-realization and liberation.

6. Enhances Core Strength

The core is the center of your body, comprising your spine, hips, and abs. These are the muscles that make it possible for us to sit up straight, breathe deeply, and walk with fluidity and balance.

Solid core muscles are vital for carrying out routine activities— from getting out of bed, bending over to fix your shoelace, and picking stuff up. Their function is more important if you're an athlete. Weak core muscles impair your strength and hinder your capacity to bend or extend your body. Worst of all, they contribute to lower back pain and muscular injury.

Hatha Yoga is one of the most powerful methods to develop strength in the body's deep core muscles. Building strength in the deep core will help maintain our spine healthy and mobile and help us do other physical exercises longer and more effectively without feeling exhausted or breathless.

Hatha Yoga improves your core muscles since it requires long-holding postures that stimulate muscles like your abdominals and glutes. Plank Pose and Warrior I are some poses that reinforce the core muscles, like the muscles in the abdomen, sides, pelvis, and back.

It could be a suitable choice for those who like to improve

their core but cannot perform higher-intensity activities such as running or weightlifting, such as older adults or individuals with some disabilities.

A 2015 analysis of Chinese adults showed that a 12-week Hatha Yoga curriculum has beneficial results on many fitness aspects, including cardio endurance, muscle strength and agility, and flexibility. Another research indicates that just 21 days of Hatha Yoga practice will contribute to improvements in core muscle strength and balance.

7. Helps Cure Inflammation and Inflammatory Disorders

There has been a considerable amount of scientific interest in Hatha Yoga lately owing to indications that it can help to minimize chronic inflammation, which can lead to a broad variety of diseases, including asthma, cardiac disease, diabetes, and cancer.

8. Hatha Yoga Lets You Have a Better Night's Sleep

Yoga is essentially a systematic cultivation of relaxation and peace of mind, so it is reasonable that it will help to improve sleep. Some researchers claim that it is great for improving sleep because it promotes mindful breathing and meditation, which will help calm your mind and body before you go to bed.

It has recently been found that Hatha Yoga significantly enhances the production of melatonin, one of the most significant sleep-regulating hormones. Also, doing Hatha Yoga will reduce your cortisol levels, a hormone that relates to your sleep cycle. Low cortisol levels are a sign to your body that it's time to sleep, so doing yoga before bed will make you fall asleep quicker.

A study reported in 2013 looked at three specific findings on the impact of Hatha Yoga on sleep patterns. The research used various lengths of yoga practice—some yoga courses lasted as long as 7 weeks, and others lasted 6 months.

The study has shown that practicing yoga in both researches has made people fall asleep quicker and increased their overall quality of sleep. Populations reported as receiving sleep benefits from yoga include cancer patients, elderly adults, people with arthritis, pregnant women, and women with menopause symptoms.

9. Decreases Anxiety and Stress

Although Hatha Yoga can be physically demanding, it can also help you calm and heal. This is because practicing yoga impacts the nervous and endocrine systems, which regulate body functions such as the production of hormones and adjustments in blood pressure.

When you get stressed or anxious, both your cortisol levels and your blood pressure increase. However, a report released in 2017 showed that people who performed a Hatha Yoga session before performing a difficult task had lower levels of cortisol and lower blood pressure than people who did not. Participants who practiced Hatha Yoga mentioned feeling more confident about their work in a challenging task.

It has also been found to reduce the production of stress-related hormones such as cortisol and activate the Parasympathetic Nervous System, the body's rest and regenerate phase.

So, the natural way to avoid stress and anxiety is to turn up on a yoga mat and do some Hatha Yoga poses. Every Hatha Yoga pose guides individuals to peace of mind and positivity.

10. Results in Healthy Glowing Skin

The Hatha Yoga Sat-Kriya leads to the thorough purification of the body. In addition, poses act as detoxifying agents at some stages, removing toxins and providing an inner glow, lustrous skin, and a rosy glow.

Here's how Hatha Yoga leaves the skin healthy and glowing.

• It releases stress, which is a primary trigger of premature aging, lack of elasticity, breakouts, and an exhausted face.

• It enhances the skin tone as it stimulates the supply of blood to the nerves below the face.

• Distribution of blood also prevents a dull complexion.

• It prevents pimples and acne from breaking out as it flushes away the pollutants.

• It stimulates the facial muscles and facilitates the supply of blood to the skin, delaying wrinkles and fine lines.

• Finally, it boosts the shine by supplying vital nutrients to the skin.

11. Improves Joint Flexibility and Mobility

As we age, it becomes more necessary to retain a healthy range of motion in the body so that we can sustain an energetic, active lifestyle in old age. When you're not working your joints to their maximum range of motion, they start to stiffen up and restrict your mobility. Many injuries to the joints, particularly the hips and knees, are triggered by repeated strain that can be directly attributed to tightness and diminished mobility in the muscles of the legs and back.

Hatha Yoga poses work your joints in several directions, enhancing mobility and flexibility. Both by lengthening and strengthening these muscles and by helping to break down the adhesions in the connective tissue around them, daily yoga practice may help relieve the strain from the joints.

Numerous researches show that just one 90-minute yoga session a week substantially improved joint mobility, particularly in the spine, of women between 50-70 years of age. Researchers also prescribe Hatha Yoga for older adults to improve the range of motion in their joints.

12. Lubricates the Joints

Hatha Yoga efficiently operates on various body joints to help them reach their maximum range of motion. In a sedentary lifestyle, the joints are not functioning to their maximum potential. As a result, they get stiffer. So do boost your joint strength with Hatha Yoga.

13. Treats Multiple Sclerosis

Yoga has been shown to have short-term impacts on mood and fatigue in people with multiple sclerosis, but has not been shown to influence muscle function, cognitive function, or quality of life.

14. Relieves Neck Pain

A 2019 meta-analysis, covering 10 studies and a total of 686 participants, showed that Hatha Yoga can minimize discomfort and pressure in the neck while also enhancing the range of motion.

15. It Enhances the Quality of Prana

Pranayama is fundamental to the practice of Hatha Yoga. The 'Pranamaya Kosha' or the 'Energy Sheath' is our essential core. It is responsible for all bodily processes, such as absorption, excretion, blood pressure, nerve impulses, and body movements. Pranayamas are specially crafted to boost our vital energy, or Prana, and to nourish the body and mind by increasing the life span. Pranayama enhances our energy intake, decreases the carbon dioxide content in our blood, enhances the body's self-healing abilities, and enhances our lifespan. It eradicates imbalances in all our physiological processes, minimizes anxiety and hypertension, and corrects hormonal imbalances.

The prana is specifically related to both body and mind since this sheath is sandwiched between the 'Annamaya Kosha' (physical body) and the 'Manomaya Kosha' (mental body). Thus, the impact of pranayama is observed both on the body and the mind. As the Prana is regulated, the mind is operated automatically. This method is used by yogis to hold the mind still. Pranayama can minimize the fluctuations of the mind (also called 'Vrittis' in Sanskrit). It may ease stresses and anxieties and therefore aid as a preparatory practice for meditation.

16. Strengthens Spine Health

Many of our nerves are branching out of the spine, linking the different organ systems to the brain. It is claimed that if the spine is stiff, nerve impulses cannot pass freely across the body, and internal organs become weakened and disease-prone. If you keep your spine supple, your nerves will stay healthy and your well-being will be preserved.

In a sedentary lifestyle, spinal health is frequently neglected, resulting in various health issues, the most frequent of which is back pain. Hatha Yoga poses for beginners such as Cobra Pose, Plank Pose, and Upward-Facing Dog relaxes the spinal muscles and helps tone the spinal muscles.

Several types of studies have shown that the success of Hatha Yoga poses along with its variants and adjustments are potent in the treatment of symptoms of lower back pain and the avoidance of impairment associated with this disorder. This natural science is particularly successful in managing back pain and offering long-lasting relief.

An analysis of the studies released in 2016 suggested that Hatha Yoga can be as successful as other non-drug therapies in the treatment of low back pain and might be stronger than normal methods.

17. It Promotes Balance and Improves the Posture

The advantage of Hatha Yoga in improving posture is very

appealing.

As we mature, our sense of freedom and stability is closely related to our sense of harmony and equilibrium. By consistently fine-tuning the body's supporting muscles and testing our spacial awareness with balancing poses, Hatha Yoga is a successful way to create sustainable balance and natural mobility.

Hatha Yoga poses will boost your ability to realize where you're in space—that's your balance and spacial awareness. Good balance prevents you from getting clumsy and potentially slipping and injuring yourself as you hit an icy street or change terrain. You also stand upright and appear more confident when you possess balance and proprioception.

18. Builds Stronger Immunity

Poor diet, lack of sleep, elevated stress, contaminants, and several medicines have a serious effect on the immune system. With a poor immune system, we are vulnerable to many pathogens and diseases. Hatha Yoga aims to improve the immune system.

When you contract and stretch your muscles, move your organs around, and get in and out of your yoga postures, you improve the supply of blood and lymph throughout the body. This helps distribute antibodies and white blood cells to fight off bacteria or foreign pathogens, kill cancer cells, and dispose of toxic waste materials for cell function.

It also helps the lymphatic system which defends the body from illness and infection. In addition, it reduces stress that adversely impacts the immune system. Hatha Yoga also keeps the level of inflammation in check to combat immune system disorders.

Some of the best yoga poses to boost the immune system are Wide-Legged Forward Fold, Headstand, Handstand, Plow Pose, and Upward Bow.

19. Relaxes the Mind and Release Stress in the Body

Yoga helps you to focus on the breath, which relaxes your mind. Whether you're attempting to find peace in a difficult pose or are looking to release stress, Hatha Yoga will help!

20. Strengthens and Tones the Body

Weight-bearing poses are held for varying lengths of time and are performed many times during practice. It's a perfect choice for functional fitness as it helps the body to be both reinforced and stretched in ways that the body normally holds on a daily basis.

21. Helps in Getting Rid of Addiction and Cravings

When our body is off track, we got all kinds of cravings. Yoga is perfect for calming our systems and helping to prevent all kinds of wacky stuff like over-sleeping, over-eating, alcohol or smoking, food cravings, PMO (P*rn Masturbation Addiction), and more!

One of the biggest advantages of Hatha Yoga is that it helps aspirants improve their willpower and regulate their cravings. It is normal because when our brains are not centered and focused, we are more inclined to engage in unhealthy food and habits. But practicing Hatha Yoga daily does a great job of calming the mind-body structure and reducing the need for external comfort.

Practicing Hatha Yoga daily, in the right way as learned by an experienced instructor, can help to suppress even intense and previously uncontrollable cravings that contribute to over-eating, over-sleeping, or over-indulgence in alcohol, sugar, and smoking.

22. You Develop an Optimistic Attitude

Hatha Yoga practices are directed at detoxifying, balancing the opposites, easing pain, and relaxing the mind which helps you feel secure and happy. When you feel good, it's easier for you to have an optimistic outlook on life.

23. Improves Oxygenation in the Body

The excess of anything is bad, the common saying goes. However, some exceptions stick out. More is good when talking about oxygenation. The practice of Headstand or inversion poses reverses the supply of blood and oxygen to every organ. This results in a larger availability of oxygen required for the proper working of the organs. Pranayama is another yogic method to increase oxygen intake for feeling fresh and active.

24. Helps during the Menopause

Yoga can alleviate the physical and psychological symptoms of menopause, including hot flashes.

25. Helps with Weight Loss

Hatha Yoga also lets you lose calories and tone your muscles for increased flexibility. According to a report, an average individual burns almost 3-6 calories per minute during yoga, accounting for 180 calories burned over one hour of class. Some yoga poses put strain on the muscles. This leads the muscles to get ripped up, but in a positive way. After the muscles are torn apart, they need resources to repair themselves; they use the energy from the fat contained in the body.

A 185-pound person will lose up to 400 calories for one hour of Hatha Yoga, whereas a 155-pound person will lose up to 300 calories. Some of the popular Hatha Yoga positions for weight reduction are Seated Forward Bend, Shoulder Stand, Warrior Pose, and Half-Moon Pose.

26. Hatha Yoga Can Improve Depression Symptoms

Experts agree that Hatha Yoga relieves stress since it works on neurotransmitters in the brain in a similar manner to antidepressants.

For example, practicing yoga raises the amounts of neurotransmitters such as serotonin and gamma-aminobutyric acid (GABA) in your brain. GABA calms the nervous system and can help soothe feelings of distress induced by stress, while serotonin balances emotions.

The 2013 review in Psychology study looked at four specific trials about how Hatha Yoga impacts the effects of depression. Data found that people who performed yoga once a week for as little as 5-weeks recorded dramatically lower scores on depression measurement surveys.

According to the 2018 report, only 12 sessions of daily Hatha Yoga practice will substantially reduce levels of anxiety and depression.

27. Results in a Calmer, Happier Mind

When your mind is stressed, you feel irritated and angry. Hatha Yoga poses help suppress stress-causing hormones and help expel harmful feelings by opening up the body parts that contain them steadily, resulting in a calmer and happier mind, which is the secret to a blissful mindset. Yoga retreats for beginners are another great way to unwind from a stressful life and enjoy harmony.

28. Helps in Kundalini Awakening

The primary aim of Hatha Yoga is to awaken the dormant Kundalini Shakti via asanas and pranayamas. This helps you bind to the vital energies that let you purify the entire body.

The different asanas, pranayamas, drishti, relaxation, and meditation performed under Hatha Yoga purify the energy centers and networks within the body, thereby awakening the Kundalini. It allows you to achieve higher stages of meditation as you open up your Chakras and Nadis (energy channels). With Kundalini active, you will attain higher consciousness.

29. It Builds Body-Mind Harmony

It's the science of alliance! Asanas, pranayama, meditation, and diet promote a balanced body-mind. When there is harmony, you feel no mental and psychical ailments but only spiritual wellness.

The practices are aimed at detoxification, balancing the opposites, easing the sufferings, and calming the mind that makes you feel healthy and happy. When you feel good, it is easier for you to adopt a positive attitude toward life. When there is happiness, you don't experience physical and psychological ills, but only mental well-being.

30. Promotes Mindfulness and Spiritual Growth

A peaceful mind is a requirement for meditation and higher practice of Samadhi, which contributes to spiritual growth. Fluctuations of the mind may be eliminated through Hatha Yoga practices such as Trataka (concentrating on a point or object) and pranayama. Yoga lets one cope with issues in life with awareness, stably and calmly, without responding to circumstances. It helps to establish healthy relationships in society.

31. You Achieve a Peaceful Mind

Hatha Yoga includes a series of asanas and pranayama rituals that regulate main stress indicators, such as high blood pressure so that the body can relax and the mind can heal. And the mediation methods are avowed for their magical ability to maintain the fluctuations of the mind (Chitta Vritti Nirodha).

32. It Adds to General Well-Being

Hatha Yoga is the road to physiological, psychological, and mental well-being. Its numerous activities make a powerful contribution to relieving the challenges of the body, mind, and soul with far-reaching effects.

Daily Hatha Yoga Practice strengthens various facets of physical, mental, and spiritual life by honoring practitioners with a productive and balanced body, mind, and soul. By supplying a healthy body, a calm mind, heightened consciousness, improved focus, and aligned energies, this yoga style guarantees the absolute and complete well-being of the practitioners.

It is claimed that the practice of Hatha Yoga would enable one to attain these symptoms: Natural appetite, healthy digestion, sound sleep, proper functioning of the different organs of the body, proper pulsation, timely removal of waste, interest in fulfilling one's duties, and happiness of mind.

I highly insist that you should practice Hatha Yoga to fill your body with healthy stimuli, mind with unbound peace, and heart with absolute positivity. Make Hatha Yoga a part of your life to live in absolute harmony and balance.

33. You Attain Inner Bliss

In Sanskrit, the word for perfect health is "Swasthya," meaning 'established or centered on one's inner self.' Yoga will certainly help us establish ourselves in this inner paradise, which is our pure essence.

'Anandamaya Kosha,' or 'Bliss Sheath,' is the innermost aspect of our being. Bliss is the center of the soul. In the Scriptures, the soul is defined as 'Sat-Chit-Ananda or Being-Consciousness-Bliss.' This bliss is experienced in deep sleep. The pleasure that we get during our day-to-day lives is just a lower manifestation of this inner paradise.

It's hard to speak about how Hatha Yoga will help your bliss sheath. It can't, in fact. Bliss is our inner nature, our pure essence! You don't have to do anything to make life better. But you will definitely erase the barriers that hinder you from enjoying this inner bliss. External interactions and the turbulence of life distort and steal away this inherent peace. Hatha Yoga can reduce these disturbances, grant us the resilience of mind, prana, and body, and give us back our sense of well-being.

THINGS YOU NEED TO
KNOW BEFORE STARTING

I f a session is Hatha, it usually implies that you'll get a gentle introduction to the most basic yoga postures. You certainly won't sweat in a Hatha Yoga session, but you'll end up leaving the session feeling longer, looser, and calmer.

Hatha Yoga is considered a perfect yoga for relaxation and mindfulness development. Practice also has lessons for calming down (like the end relaxation and Trataka Meditation), focusing on the body, and progressing without jumping from one pose to the next. There are several things to be learned from everyday Hatha practice that will benefit both the mind and your body.

Unlike the energizing and fast-moving Vinyasa Yoga, Hatha Yoga is deliberately slower and strongly breathing-based. It's always the perfect place for beginners to have their feet immersed in yoga, yet Hatha is great for everybody.

But as with the start of every physical activity, a mixture of enthusiasm and nervousness can be encountered, and beginning a new yoga practice is no different. Therefore, to make you feel more at ease, this section will cover choices on when and where to practice yoga, the essentials, what to expect in the session, and tips for progress in your practice.

The following is a list of tips to help guide you on what kind of environment, time, and items you would need for your Hatha Yoga session. Also, how you can make the best out of your yoga session and some tips for beginners.

When and Where to Practice Hatha Yoga?

When to Practice?

Hatha Yoga should be practiced early in the morning. But if you can't, it is fine to practice at other times of the day as well. However, here are some reasons to motivate you towards practicing in the early morning hours.

• Early morning is called 'Brahmamuhurta' in Sanskrit. It means 'The Divine Time.' This is the time of the day when the spiritual energy on our lovely planet is at its highest.

• The air at this time is fresh and contains the greatest amount of Prana (Cosmic Life Force).

• The mind is also fresh and unburdened with the worries of everyday life. This will help in the practice of focus and meditation.

• This is the time of day when you are least likely to be distracted by the hustle and bustle of everyday life.

• The stomach is empty, which is necessary before practicing many of the asanas and pranayamas.

Where to Practice Hatha Yoga?

All that is required to perform Hatha Yoga is a flat floor and enough space to stretch out. A well-ventilated area is ideal to promote healthy breathing. Practicing outdoors is fine as well, although in direct sunlight it may become too warm due to the energetic pranayamas and asanas.

Items You'll Need

1. **Hatha Yoga Guide:** Optional; if you're already familiar with the sequence, you don't need to have a class recording. Instead, just come to your sacred place and practice.

2. Yoga Mat: Yoga mats are essential to provide a non-slip surface for standing poses. Choose a supportive mat that has a thickness of at least 5 mm.

3. Candles: There's something special about the candles. It might just be the bright glow and the ambient flicker of the flames. It's a tradition—candles have been used as a sign of life, purity, and goodness in religious rituals for hundreds of years. The lighting of the candle is a sign of our highest intentions, best wishes, and prayers. Placing candles throughout the room not only adds warmth but also adds an ethereal feel to the training.

NOTE: Be sure that the candles are away from flammable materials and are set on safe surfaces.

4. Essential Oils: Essential oils are potent natural remedies because they contain the beneficial curing properties of the plant. Each oil has a distinctive odor and vibration that can enhance the body's emotional and physical experiences.

When oils come into contact with the skin, they are incorporated into the tissues that influence the body as a whole. Furthermore, by our sense of scent, the oils are connected to the portion of our brains correlated with sentiment and memory, which will affect mood and mind. Daily practice combining yoga and essential oils is a great complement to our self-care routines.

5. Clothing:

Loose, comfortable clothes should be worn. Choose a tank top or t-shirt that moves with you, but it's a good idea to have a sweatshirt or blanket during the relaxation period. Any comfortable bottom (shorts, capris, or pants) in cotton or stretched fabric that breathes and allows movement is great.

6. Blocks: Though blocks are not mandatory in Hatha Yoga, you can use them as a common accessory, especially if you aren't versatile or need a prop for support in certain poses.

How to Get the Most Out of an At-Home Hatha Yoga Session?

1. Choose a Quiet, Soothing Space

It's a lot easier to do yoga if you're in an environment that calms and motivates you to do so. Try to find a space where it's peaceful and quiet, with as much area around you within which you can perform poses without hitting anything.

Practice at a time when distractions are minimal, so if you're worried that babies, pets, or spouses could disturb you, let everyone know that you need this specific minute of quiet time. Switch your phone to silent and leave it out of reach. Light the candle, dim the lamps, remove any mess, and get ready to practice.

2. Try Organizing Your Space

Calmness is improved if the environment where you practice is as stress-free as possible. The room should be clean, warm, and softly illuminated. Before you begin, be conscious of what resources you need for your entire session. Have all your essentials ready—water bottle, practice guide, and blocks—near your mat in an organized manner.

3. Consider Warm-Up

It's always advised to do some warm-ups before you perform various asanas. The following are ideal for warming up: Pelvis Rotations, Spinal Flex, Neck Rolls, Side Twists, Side Bends, Shoulder Shrugs, Cobra, Rock & Roll on the Spine, Alternate Leg Extension, and Cat-Cow.

Warm-up postures help you prepare for upcoming activities. You're enhancing muscle flexibility, loosening regions of the body, increasing blood supply to the extremities, and concentrating your attention on the task ahead. All-in-all, a warm-up routine is just as critical as the yoga practice itself.

NOTE: Make sure you only perform 2-3 warm-ups and define clearly the beginning of the practice.

4. Know That It's Not a Workout

Many Westerners think of Hatha Yoga as a physical workout —a workout that provides a feeling of relaxation, but also an exercise. They head to classes hoping to break the sweat and tone their bodies, and in a power or flow class, they're definitely going to. Hatha Yoga is not, though, a workout. Instead, it's a gentle form of yoga, and the aim is to work the mind, body, and soul. There are limited poses and each pose is kept for several minutes.

5. Breathe Right

To raise the coiled, invisible, serpentine energy at the bottom of your spine, yogis use special breathing exercises. These are exercises that wake the unconscious Kundalini whether they're energizing or relaxing.

Our breathing is normally unconscious. You may never care about an appropriate breathing technique or breathing quality. However, breathing techniques can offer several advantages, for example, relaxation or increased energy.

(We'll explore the various breathing techniques/pranayamas of Hatha Yoga ahead.)

6. Practice Regularly

We feel tired in body and soul and our capacity to cope with the struggles of our lives is decreased when our energy levels are low. Hatha Yoga allows us, with daily practice, to develop a deep core of Prana or life force, and to develop a reservoir of love within. We can rely on this reservoir to have the power to fulfill everyday life requirements.

7. Keep It Simple

Yoga should always be suited to one's state of health; that is, a shorter and easier routine should be practiced when a person is tired.

8. Be Comfortable

In yoga, nothing should be uncomfortable. Be sure that in your clothes you can breathe and move effortlessly. Avoid anything that makes you uncomfortable.

9. Avoid Noise

If you're in town or in a busy neighborhood, keep your windows closed to prevent noise. But if you live in a remote place near nature, consider cracking a window and welcoming the sounds of nature to your house.

10. Always Relax with Savasana at the End

It's very important to allow your body the time to recover after a yoga session in Savasana. The nervous system requires time to assimilate the benefits it has gained in practice.

Just as it is important to warm up the muscles at the start of the session, cooling down is just as vital to calm down the rejuvenated muscles at the end of the session. Thus, one should always finish the yoga session with Savasana. This asana is designed to help the body relax and restore breathing and increased circulation back to normal.

Some Beginners Tips

1. Always practice after taking a shower and empty your bladder and bowels.

2. Never practice on a full stomach.

3. Always listen to your body. The beauty of yoga is that if anything doesn't feel right, it's fine to get out of it. There's no "No Pain-No Gain" attitude here. It's OK not to go to the full expression of the pose, because where you are, as long as you have the correct posture, it's beneficial. What you want to do is go to the "Edge"—where you experience sensation, but not pain.

4. Do not eat any meal right after yoga. There should be a gap of at least 20-30 minutes between the practice and the meal.

5. You must not hold your breath until you are clearly instructed to do so. And always breathe from the nostrils unless otherwise instructed.

6. If you're in a class, don't compare your practice with that of another student, even the coach, or also your own (because your body varies day-to-day-sometimes in the same pose from one side to the other). Focus on your practice, breathing, and what the teacher tells you. Competition can rid you of the enjoyment of your practice and will make you attempt poses that your body is not ready for.

7. Those just starting Hatha Yoga practice often report exhaustion and soreness in the body, as yoga stretches and exercises muscles and tendons that are sometimes long-neglected. Some yogic breathing and mediations can be challenging for beginners and can induce dizziness or disorientation. Whenever this occurs, just relax and keep going as per your will. Overtime, exhaustion and soreness will be gone and you will be able to perform the various practices seamlessly.

8. If you feel weak during asanas, drink a glass of lukewarm water with honey.

HATHA YOGA POSES

There are almost 200 Hatha Yoga postures, with hundreds of variants. It's easy to look at it and get overwhelmed. But you don't have to do that. Although the start of your journey is powerful, it can be very easy.

Hatha is considered to be a gentle yoga that emphasizes static poses and is perfect for beginners. However, even though it's gentle, it can still be physically and mentally challenging.

The Hatha Yoga routine is a series of physical postures and breathing techniques. Routines can take anything from 20 minutes to 2 hours, based on the needs and skills of the practitioner.

For a traditionalist, Hatha Yoga postures are just the beginning of the process. They help to prepare the body for seated meditation practices that enable us to reach the higher limbs of yoga.

The session normally starts with a gentle warm-up (Sun Salutation), progresses to more physical poses, and concludes with a short period of meditation. Here is the rundown of a standard class:

Sun Salutation: Several Hatha classes use Sun Salutations to warm up the body and build up heat within. Sun Salutation is a flow of yoga asanas linked with breathing. They are incredibly energizing, and integrating the inhalation and exhalation with each transition generates a moving meditation, promoting stillness and concentration in the mind.

Asanas: You'll be doing standing postures, core work, balancing postures, backbends, inversions, and floor poses. The layout of the session is organized in a standardized manner to make it easier for you to get the best out of each pose. Poses vary in complexity from lying flat on the floor to physically demanding positions.

Savasana: This pose is everyone's favorite. This final pose requires you to lie on your back with your arms and legs apart, like a starfish, and to let go fully.

Savasana is an important part of the yoga practice which gives the body and mind time to rejuvenate and absorb all the positive work you have done with your body. You will usually lie here for 5-10 minutes, with your eyes closed and your body heavy on the floor. Breathing deeply in Savasana helps you to relieve stress in your body and to wake up feeling energized and nourished.

Being mindful of your breath makes it easier for your mind to stay in the current moment and helps create the framework for sitting meditation.

Pranayama: Pranayama translates to 'extension of life force.' 'Prana' means life energy or breath, and 'Ayama' means to extend. Pranayama practice prolongs the life within us and awakens our Kundalini energy.

Pranayama comprises controlled breathing techniques that have a direct impact on your nervous system and the energy of your body's life force. You would be introduced to deep breathing techniques and possibly some breathing exercises to stimulate or relax your mind and body, depending on the nature or time of the class.

Meditation: The bulk of Hatha Yoga classes conclude with a brief meditation. During this time of peaceful relaxation, you sit in Sukhasana or Lotus Pose and enjoy a relaxing meditation.

The standard Hatha Yoga class ends with participants putting their hands together in a Prayer Pose over their hearts, bowing and saying Namaste to each other and thanking God.

Warm-Up (Sun Salutation/Surya Namaskar)

Surya Namaskar has become the default beginning point to warm up in many yoga classes today. However, the edition performed in classes only targets the hip joint. I prefer to stick to the classic Surya Namaskar to warm up the body as they offer a fuller range of motion in all major joints.

Beyond being a perfect aerobic exercise, Surya Namaskar is also considered to have an overwhelmingly beneficial impact on the body and mind.

Surya Namaskar is usually performed early in the morning on an empty stomach. Besides good health, Surya Namaskar also offers an opportunity to express gratitude to the sun for sustaining life on this planet.

Benefits:

• Performing Surya Namaskar in the morning energizes the body, mind, and soul, drawing energy from the sun.

• In Hinduism and other traditions with Vedic origins, the Sun symbolizes consciousness and is often worshiped. The Surya Namaskar vinyasas are an extension of that worship, honoring the Sun's power within.

• It helps to improve cardiovascular health.

• The postures are the right blend of warm-ups and asanas.

• It helps to keep you disease-free and healthy.

• Regular practice promotes balance in the body.

• Improves blood circulation.

• Strengthens the heart.

• Tones the digestive tract.

• Stimulates abdominal muscles, respiratory system, lymphatic system, spinal nerves, and other internal organs.

• Tones the spine, neck, shoulder, arms, hands, wrist, back, and leg muscles, thereby promoting overall flexibility.

• Psychologically, it regulates the interconnectedness of body, breath, and mind, thus making you calmer and boosting your energy levels with sharpened awareness.

• It increases energy and vitality, thereby making your face glow with radiance. This helps the skin retain its firmness.

• Surya Namaskar prevents the onset of wrinkles by relieving the body and mind of stress.

• Reduces mood swings and brings more emotional stability.

• It stimulates the nervous system.

• It helps to stretch, flex, and tone the muscles.

• Sun Salutation is a great exercise to control weight loss.

• It strengthens the immune system.

• It increases cognitive function.

• It improves general health, strengthens the body, and relaxes the mind.

How to Do:

1. Tadasana (Standing Mountain Pose)

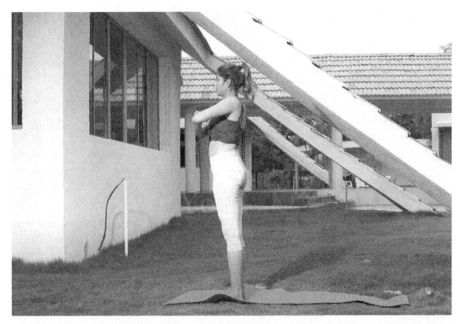

Stand with your feet hip-width apart. In Prayer Pose, bring the palms together. Relax your thumbs on the sternum and take a few breaths.

2. Urdhva Hastasana (Upward Salute)

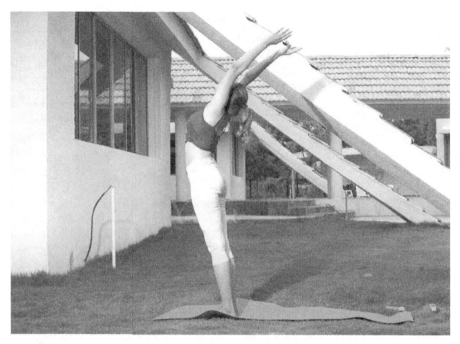

Inhale as you sweep your arms to the side and overhead. Kindly arch your back and face up toward the ceiling.

3. Uttanasana (Standing Forward Fold)

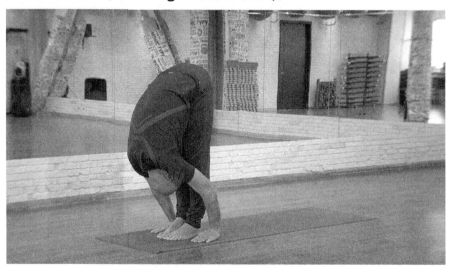

Exhale as you fold your hips forward. Bend your knees if you need to. Relax your hands beside your legs and bring your nose as close to your feet as you can.

4. Ardha Uttanasana (Half-Standing Forward Fold)

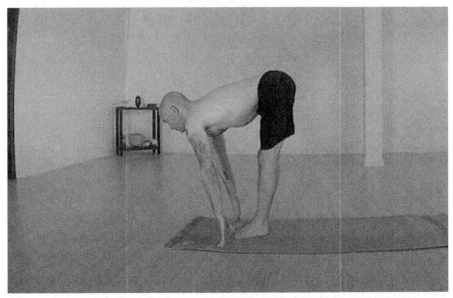

Inhale as you raise your torso halfway; lengthen your spine forward such that your back becomes flat. Your torso should be parallel to the floor. Keep your fingertips on the floor, or put them on your shins.

5. High Lunge

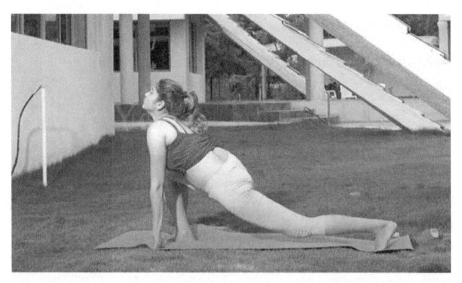

Exhale and step your left foot back into a lunge. Center your right knee over the heel, so that your shin is perpendicular to the floor, and bring your right thigh parallel to the floor. Firm your tailbone against your pelvis and press your right thigh against the resistance. Inhale and reach back through your left heel. Lengthen the torso looking up towards the ceiling. Look forward without being strained.

6. Adho Mukha Svanasana (Downward-Facing Dog Pose)

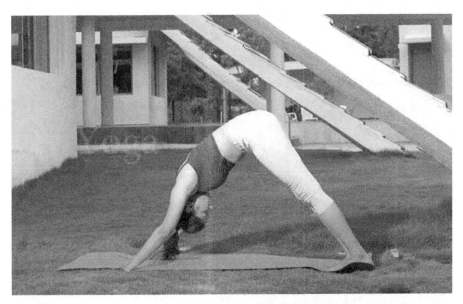

Exhale and take your left foot back. Stretch the palms and soles. Press the front of your thighs back as you press your inner hands strongly against the floor. Think that your torso is being stretched like a rubber band between your arms and legs.

7. Chaturanga Dandasana (Four-Limbed Staff Pose)

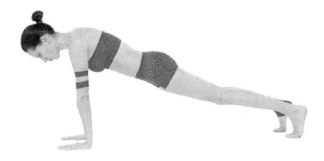

Inhale and leap into Plank Pose (High Push-Up Pose) with your hands under your shoulders and your legs hip-distance apart. Exhale as you drop your body to the floor. Keep your elbows tucked into your sides. If you need to, come to your knees for Half-Chaturanga. Otherwise, leave your legs straight and go back through your heels.

8. Ashtanga Namaskara (Salute with Eight Parts or Points)

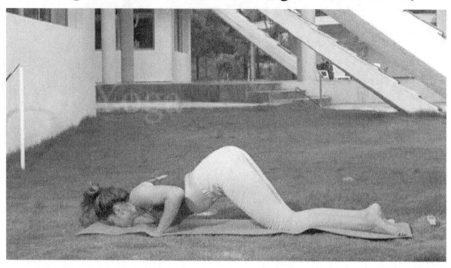

Continue exhaling as you gently bring your knees to the floor. Take your hips back slightly, slide forward, and rest your chest and chin on the floor. Raise your hips a little. The two hands, two feet, two knees, the chest, and the chin (eight parts of the body) should touch the floor.

9. Urdhva Mukha Svanasana (Upward-Facing Dog Pose)

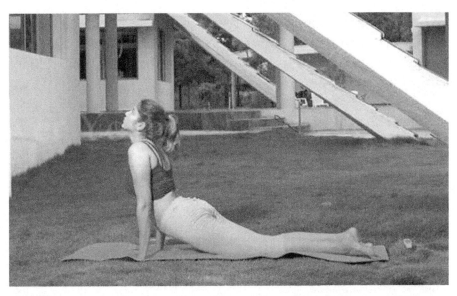

Inhale as you pull your chest forward and straighten your arms. Drag your shoulders back and lift your heart to the ceiling. Push through the tops of your feet, raise your thighs off the floor, and keep your leg muscles fully engaged. Keep your elbows tucked in toward your sides.

10. Adho Mukha Svanasana (Downward-Facing Dog Pose)

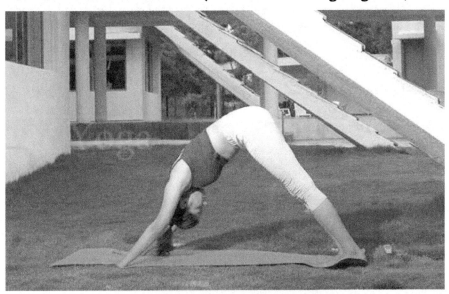

Exhale and once again stretch the palms and soles. Press the front of your thighs back as you press your inner hands strongly against the floor. Think that your torso is being stretched like a rubber band between your arms and legs.

11. High Lunge

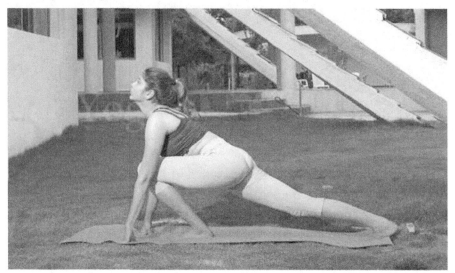

Inhale and bring your left leg upfront. Center your left knee over the heel, so that your shin is perpendicular to the floor, and bring your left thigh parallel to the floor. Firm your tailbone against your pelvis and press your left thigh against the resistance. Lengthen the torso looking up towards the ceiling. Look forward without being strained.

12. Ardha Uttanasana (Half-Standing Forward Fold)

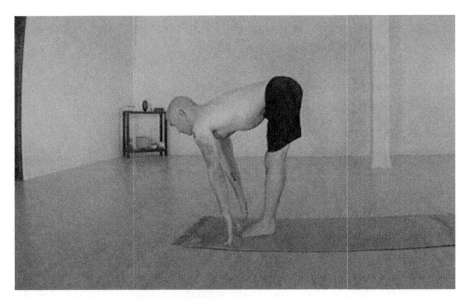

Exhale as you bring your right leg to your left leg. Inhale as you step or leap between your hands. Raise your torso halfway, lengthening your spine forward such that your back is flat. Your torso should be parallel to the floor. Keep your fingertips on the floor, or put them on your shins.

13. Uttanasana (Standing Forward Fold)

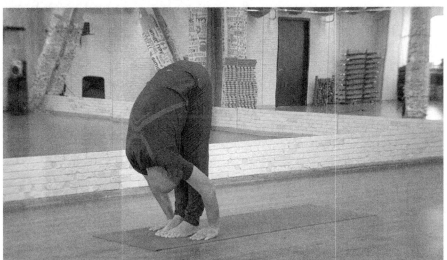

Exhale as you fold the torso over your thighs. Bend your knees if you need to. Relax your hands beside your feet and bring your nose to your feet as long as you can.

14. Urdhva Hastasana (Upward Salute)

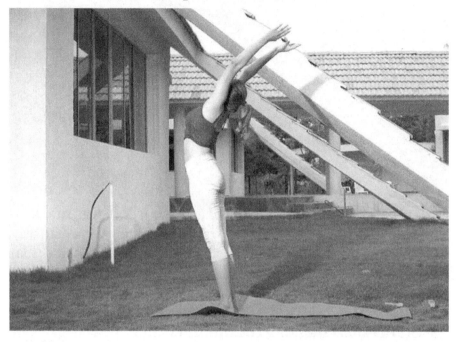

Inhale as you reach your arms out to the side and stretch out once again. Kindly stretch your back and look up toward the ceiling.

15. Tadasana (Mountain Pose)

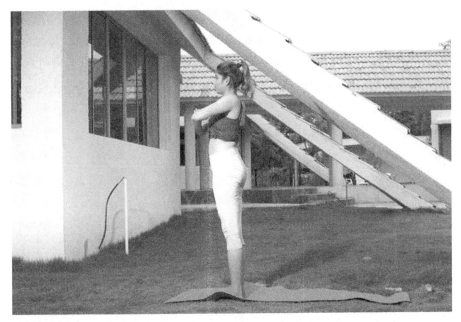

Exhale as you come back into Mountain Pose. Bring your hands into the Prayer Pose. Rest your thumbs on your sternum.

Contradictions:

• Heart patients should consult their doctor before performing this sequence.

• If you have back issues, you must perform Sun Salutation under the supervision of your yoga instructor.

• People with high blood pressure problems should avoid this sequence.

• Arthritis contributes to the stiffness of the knee and therefore hinders movement. Since Surya Namaskar includes knee motions, you must be careful if you are an arthritis patient.

• Persons suffering from hernia must always refrain from performing Sun Salutation.

• If you have a serious wrist injury, you may skip this yoga sequence.

• Pregnant women should not perform Sun Salutation because it places weight on the back and abdominal areas, causing damage to both the mother and the child.

• Women must also avoid Surya Namaskar during their periods.

Timing: 3-5 rounds

Hatha Yoga Asanas

1. Simhasana (Lion Pose)

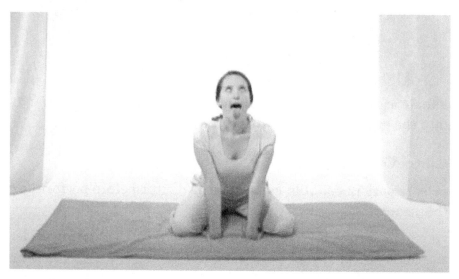

Sacred ancient scriptures such as Gheranda Samhita have revealed that this specific asana is the 'Destroyer of Diseases.' It encourages independence and self-reliance. Simhasana triggers all three major Bandhas—Mula, Jalandhara, and Uddiyana.

The Simhasana is called as it represents a roaring lion in its final state. This asana needs the body and the face to function toward invoking the deep roar of the lion. This is a fairly relaxed asana that anyone can do. It is not a common posture; the advantages are distinct from those of the other asanas. Have a peek at what this asana has to offer you.

Benefits:

• In the yogic text of Gheranda Samhita, Simhasana is defined as the destroyer of all diseases.

• Simhasana preserves good health throughout the head region —ears, nose, throat, and eyes. Practicing it in front of the rising sun makes it more beneficial.

• According to the Hatha Yoga text, Hatha Yoga Pradeepika, Simhasana helps execute three bandhas or locks, namely Mula Bandha, Uddiyana Bandha, and Jalandhara Bandha.

• Simhasana effectively decreases emotional stress and reduces anger.

• Relieves stress in the chest and facial muscles and helps the face appear youthful. Steady breathing in this posture supports both the chest and the abdomen.

• Useful for people who are shy, sometimes anxious, or introverted by nature.

• Exercises the muscles of the face and neck, holding the skin tight.

• Beneficial to those who shutter.

• The practitioner gains a lovely, sonorous voice. It helps to overcome several voice-based issues.

• Develops a deep, strong accent.

• Useful for someone with halitosis.

• This asana is said to eradicate deficiencies in the throat, nose, mouth, and ears. Poor breath is also eliminated.

How to Do:

1. Distance your knees as much as you can.

2. The toes on both legs must meet each other, much like they do

in Vajrasana.

3. Shift the body forward slightly. Place your palms between your knees.

4. Turn your wrists out so that your fingertips point towards the body. Hold your arms straight.

5. Gently arch the back, transferring the weight of the body to the wrists. Shift your head back comfortably.

6. Shut your eyes and calm your body in this position to feel comfortable for a moment.

7. Now open your eyes and concentrate on the center of your eyebrows. Inhale gently and deeply.

8. Open your mouth and draw your tongue out to your chin as far as you can.

9. As you exhale from your mouth, make a sound of 'Aaah' coming out of your throat.

10. Shut the mouth following exhalation and normally inhale. Relax the body in the final position.

11. You should replicate this process 3-5 times. One can even shift the tongue from side to side when making the sound 'Aaah.'

Drishti: Set your eyes on the spot between the eyebrows (Third Eye Chakra).

Contradictions:

• Avoid focusing on the Third Eye if it makes you feel dizzy. Practice this just for a few seconds and gradually during the practice.

• People with weak wrists can practice Simhasana sitting in Vajrasana.

• Don't exert yourself when making the sound. Aim to keep it clear and steady.

Timing: 1-3 minutes

2. Ardha Matsyendrasana (Half-Fish Pose)

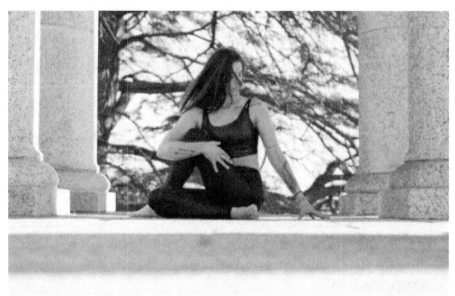

It is helpful to warm up your hips for this most freeing, balancing, and energizing of seated twists. One of the greatest things about yoga is that it puts you in positions you rarely do in the normal course of your day. Moving in different ways accesses places where you didn't even realize you were holding stress. This is true of deep twists, such as Half-Lord of the Fishes.

Benefits:

• It creates balance in the spine and on the left and right sides of the body.

• It compresses and extends the spine from bottom to top.

• It twists and rinses the spine.

• It strengthens and enhances the elasticity, flexibility, circulation, and nutrition of the spinal nerves, veins, and tissues.

• It relieves pain in the lower back.

• It increases the flexibility of the hip and back joints.

• It stretches the muscles of the chest, upper back, and outer thigh.

• It advances digestion and removes flatulence by rinsing the abdominal organs.

• It opens the shoulder joint.

• It realigns the vertebral column, easing conditions such as scoliosis, kyphosis, and lordosis.

• It increases the supply of spinal nerves, veins, and tissues.

• It calms the nervous system.

• It's the only posture that twists the spine from top to bottom at the same time helps prevent slipped discs, scoliosis, arthritis, and rheumatism.

• It relieves lethargy and tension.

• It helps to cure nausea and dizziness.

• It maintains youth by improving spine flexibility.

• It helps lumbago and rheumatism in the spine.

• It improves digestion and prevents flatulence in the intestines.

• It firms your abdomen, thighs, and buttocks.

• Improves postural and body awareness

How to Do:

1. T-Bend the right leg on the floor so the right foot meets the left buttock; bend the left knee to bring the left leg up and down the right leg; line the left heel up to reach the right knee.

2. Ensure that the right knee and both buttocks remain on the

floor throughout the pose.

3. Position your left hand up behind your back, next to your tailbone, to support your body weight forward and lifted throughout the pose.

4. Inhale while stretching the right arm towards the right ear.

5. Exhale while dragging the right arm over the left knee to hold the right kneecap firmly.

6. Inhale as the spine is raised.

7. Exhale as you turn your head over your left shoulder, and twist your shoulders and torso to the left.

8. Deepen the twist by doing the following:

• Push your right elbow on your left knee; extend your left hand behind your back all the way around to hold your right thigh or hip.

9. Breath normally and work towards a deeper twist, especially during exhalation.

NOTE: Keep the abdominal muscles engaged to support the spine, and use the core strength to avoid twisting the rounded, unsupported spine.

10. Perform lifting as you twist.

11. Lift the abdomen out of the pelvis and lift the upper body towards the ceiling.

12. Work your shoulders down and away from your ears.

13. Breathe, keep the pose for 20 seconds, and then unwind.

14. Repeat this pose on the right by twisting to the right.

Drishti: Keep your gaze soft or you can even close your eyes.

Contradictions:

• People with severe back or neck pain should practice with

patience and close observation.

• Anyone with slipped disc should avoid posing this completely.

• Those with internal organ disorders can find this to be challenging and painful.

• Pregnant women should avoid it because it can push the fetus.

Timing: 20-60 seconds, on each side

3. Bhujangasana (Cobra Pose)

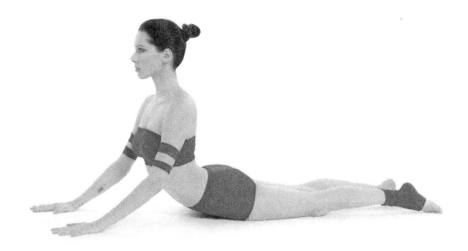

Everyone loves Cobra Pose or Bhujangasana. Great for stretching and strengthening the core, this pose can help prevent back pain. Cobra Pose is one of those nice yoga postures, which is easy to do and gives many important health benefits. It is not only great for the health and flexibility of your back and spine but is also excellent for regulating your digestive system and toning other abdominal organs.

According to ancient yogic texts, this posture heals the ill body and awakens Kundalini, the divine cosmic spirit that promotes self-realization.

Benefits:

• Activates the Heart Chakra.

• In advanced stages, the Kundalini Shakti awoke.

• Massages all the digestive organs, enhancing both absorption and elimination.

• Works on balancing both the Manipura Chakra and the Svadhishthana Chakra.

• Works on all the nerve junctions that lie along the spine, as well as the big psychic channels that run across the spinal cord.

• Works to enhance the function of ovaries and reproductive glands.

• Acts on thyroid and parathyroid glands and Vishuddhi Chakra.

• Opens up the Heart Chakra that encourages softness of character.

• Great for vision improvement and optical nerve toning.

• It relieves menstrual problems, such as back pain, cramping, and irregularity.

• It cures a lack of appetite.

• It helps to correct posture.

• It strengthens the focus.

• It promotes circulation and proper alignment of the back and abdomen.

• It reduces symptoms of PMS and helps in proper digestion.

• It develops a precise awareness of the body.

• It prevents and cures back pain and herniated vertebral discs.

• It increases spinal strength and flexibility

• It helps prevent lower back pain and helps cure lumbago,

rheumatism, and spinal arthritis.

• It increases the functioning of the liver and spleen.

• It strengthens the deltoids, trapezius, and triceps.

How to Do:

1. Lie down on the belly.

2. Put palms flat on the floor directly underneath the shoulders, fingertips in line with the tops of the shoulders.

3. Hold the legs together and keep them stretched down and back.

4. Pull your shoulders down and keep your elbows close to your ribs.

5. Use the strength of the spine and legs instead of the arms for the next step (it's not a push-up).

6. Inhale, look up to the ceiling, and arch your head and torso until the belly button just touches the floor.

8. Keep your gaze slightly raised and avoid supporting your body weight with your hands.

9. Keep your elbows tight to the sides of your body and relax your face.

10. Hold the pose for 20 seconds while breathing normally.

11. Lower chin to the floor.

Drishti: While performing this pose, focus your gaze upwards, towards the ceiling.

Contradictions:

• Stop doing Bhujangasana if you are pregnant, have fractured ribs or wrists, or have just undergone abdominal surgery, such as a hernia.

• Avoid Bhujangasana if you have Carpal Tunnel Syndrome.

• Perform Cobra Pose under the supervision of a yoga instructor if you have suffered from chronic diseases or spinal disorders in the past.

Timing: 20-60 seconds

4. Salabhasana (Locust Pose)

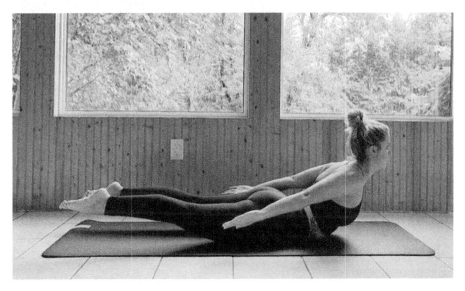

Salabhasana or Locust Pose is a back bent that appears like a grasshopper. Practice it in the morning on an empty stomach or in the evening following 4 to 6 hours of the last meal. Salabhasana is a beginner-level yoga asana.

Locust Pose strengthens and helps stabilize the 1st chakra (Root Chakra or Muladhara) found at the base of your spine. It helps keep you grounded and improves your feelings of safety and security. The imbalances in this chakra can trigger anxiety or fear.

Benefits:

• All back extensions bring awareness to the front body.

• It encourages focus and dedication.

• It targets the top of the back.

• It boosts circulation.

• It provides flexibility and tones the spinal muscles.

• It invigorates the muscles of the arm and back.

• Lifting the front body, particularly the chest cavity, helps develop courage and mental strength.

• It strengthens the shoulders, breasts, elbows, wrists, and spine.

• It develops core strength.

• It reverses common problems related to repetitive stress in the forearms, hands, and elbows.

• It increases circulation in the leg and stops and reduces varicose veins.

• It reinforces the upper back, arms, fingers, hamstrings, and calves.

• It helps with back or spinal disorders such as gout, slipped discs, and sciatica.

• It helps with tennis elbows and is also good for toning buttocks and hip rotators.

• It's excellent for firming buttocks and hips.

• Aids in Body Balance.

• In our practice, we begin to lose patience and dedication; backbends help to add vitality back to the yoga practice.

How to Do:

1. Start lying on your stomach with your arms extended down by your sides, and palms facing up. Allow your forehead to rest on the floor naturally. Press the tailbone to the ground.

2. Lift your head, chest, and arms off the floor on the inhale.

3. Lift your legs off the ground on the exhale.

4. Look down, so the front and back of your neck are the same lengths. Roll the shoulder blades onto your back. Reach back through your fingertips and toes.

5. Feel your inner thighs lift your legs off the ground. Drop the tailbone to the ground.

6. Hold for 30-60 seconds and then drop in belly-down Savasana.

Drishti: Nasagre (Tip of the nose).

Contradictions:

• Must not perform this pose if you're having headaches at the moment.

• Also avoid this pose if you have recent or chronic back or neck injuries.

• Always work within your range of limitations and abilities.

• Talk to a doctor before practicing it if you have any medical concerns.

Timing: 20-60 seconds

5. Halasana (Plow Pose)

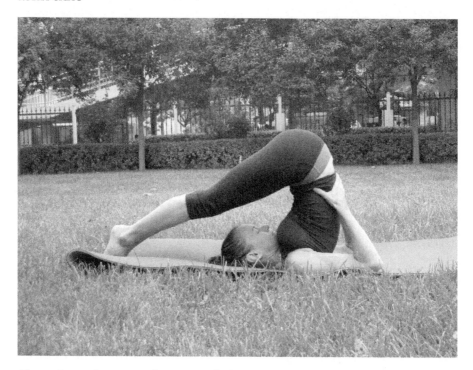

Plow Pose in yoga is one of those postures that coils you up and makes you appear as twisted as a pretzel. It provides many advantages, like relaxing the spine and soothing the mind, but it is frequently discouraged by practitioners and certain instructors because of the strain it places on the cervical spine and neck.

Plow Pose improves circulation, endurance, and vitality, and therefore prepares the body for relaxing and meditation.

Benefits:

• Massages the internal organs.

• Plow Pose helps you sleep better.

• Enhances the functionality of the spinal nerves by creating a strain on the normally sympathetic nerves of the neck, thereby improving the functionality of the Sympathetic Nervous System.

• Good for dyspepsia.

• Stimulates the digestive organs.

• Helps with constipation.

• Revitalizes the spleen.

• Promotes the production of insulin.

• Strengthens the pancreas, liver, and kidneys.

• Strengthens the abdominal muscles.

• Assists with back pain.

• Plow Pose relieves stress.

• Promotes blood circulation.

• Controls the thyroid gland and thus the energy intake of the body.

• Strengthens the immune system.

How to Do:

1. Lie flat on your back with your arms close to your body, your palms facing up.

2. Inhale and lift your legs while tightening your abdominal muscles. Take the legs to an angle of 90°.

3. Use your hands to support your hips as you raise them off the floor.

4. Now put your legs to an inclination of 180° so that your toes meet the ground behind your head.

5. Keep this posture for 10 seconds to up to a minute and focus on your breathing. Breathe gently and peacefully.

6. To get out of the pose, exhale and put the legs back to their starting position slowly and controlled.

Drishti: Focus your gaze on your navel or the tip of your nose.

Contradictions:

• For glaucoma practitioners (an eye disease that damages the optic nerve) inversions such as a Headstand, Shoulder Stand, and Handstand are generally prohibited. These poses further intensify the already too-intensive strain on the optic nerve.

• Avoid doing this asana with:

- Diarrhea
- Menstruation
- Neck injury

• If you have elevated blood pressure and asthma, support your legs with props while you are practicing this.

• If you're breastfeeding, just do this asana if you've been doing it for a long time. Don't start practicing when you're pregnant.

• When you touch your foot to the ground, this asana becomes an advanced yoga posture. That's why you must perform this asana under the supervision of an experienced yoga instructor.

Timing: 10-60 seconds

6. Setu Bandhasana (Bridge Pose)

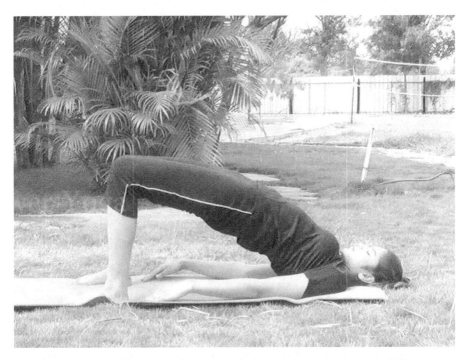

Setu Bandhasana or Bridge Pose is a common asana. This asana is named after the Sanskrit words 'Setu,' which means bridge, 'Bandha,' which means lock, and 'Asana,' which means pose. This pose resembles the structure of the bridge and is therefore named. This posture stretches your back, neck, and chest, calming your body.

The bridge is a link between two different places, which can be physical, spiritual, or psychological. By building a bridge with your body, you create a transformation-inducing structure that can get you from where you are to where you want to be.

Benefits:

• Strengthens back muscles.

• Relieves the tired back instantly.

• Gives a good stretch to the chest, neck, and spine.

• Calms the subconscious.

• Opens the lungs and eliminates concerns with the thyroid.

• Aims to boost digestion.

• It lengthens the spine and opens the chest.

• Promotes peace of mind and boosts attention.

• Helps with depression (for mild energizing when energy is low).

• Deals with general weakness.

• Helps to relieve symptoms of menopause and menstrual pain.

• Calms the brain and helps to relieve stress and mild depression.

• Stimulates the abdominal organs, lungs, and thyroid gland.

• Rejuvenates tired legs.

• Helps to relieve the symptoms of menopause.

• Reduces anxiety, fatigue, back pain, headaches, and insomnia.

• Therapeutic for asthma, elevated blood pressure, osteoporosis, and sinusitis.

How to Do:

1. To start, lie on your back.

2. Bend your knees and keep your feet separated on the floor, 10-12 inches from your pelvis, with your knees and ankles in a straight line.

3. Keep your arms beside your body, your palms facing down.

4. Inhale and steadily raise your lower back, middle back, and upper back off the floor.

5. Next, softly roll in your shoulders and touch your chest to your chin without bringing your chin down, maintaining your weight with your shoulders, arms, and feet. Feel your bottom firm up in this pose. Both legs are parallel to each other and to the floor.

6. If you want, you could interlace your fingers and press your hands to the floor to lift the torso up a bit, or you could support your back with your palms.

7. Keep your breathing normal.

7. Hold the posture for a minute or two and exhale as you gently release the pose.

Drishti: Forward or toward the nose (Nasagre).

Contradictions:

• People who have a neck injury must either completely avoid this asana or do it with doctor's consent under a professional yoga teacher.

• Pregnant women can do this asana, but not to the fullest extent possible. They must do this under the guidance of a yoga expert. If they are in their third trimester, they must do this asana with the consent of their doctor.

• If you have problems with your back, you must avoid this asana.

Timing: 1-3 minutes

7. Dhanurasana (Upward Bow)

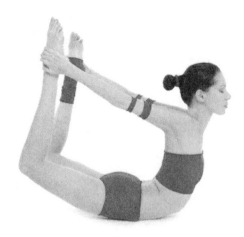

Upward Bow Pose is an intermediate stage of back-bending asana. Essentially, it is a gentle inversion that stretches the complete body, particularly the spine and abdomen, and improves the overall flexibility and strength of the body.

This asana is very useful to those who sit in front of screens for long hours, as it eliminates stress and pain from their bodies.

Benefits:

• Stretches the chest and shoulders.

• Raises energy and compensates for depression.

• Strengthens the arms and wrists, legs, hip flexors, abdomen, and spine.

• Relieves many types of low back pain.

• Great for respiratory conditions like asthma, opening the auxiliary muscles of breathing.

• Activates the thyroid and pituitary glands and helps to stabilize hormones and metabolism.

• Energizes a tired body/mind.

• Stimulates Manipura Chakra.

• Decreases discomfort in the back.

• Can improve fertility.

• Boost bone strength to help reduce osteoporosis.

• It is said to ignite all 7 chakras, maintaining all the body's functions in sync with each other.

How to Do:

1. Lie on your stomach with your feet hip-width apart and your arms by your sides, palms facing upward.

2. Bend your knees and bring your heels as close as possible to your buttocks.

3. Reach your arms backward and grasp your ankles with your hands. Make sure your fingers are pointing toward your toes.

4. Inhale deeply as you lift your chest off the ground, simultaneously kicking your feet into your hands. This action will raise your thighs and upper body off the mat.

5. Keep your gaze forward and maintain a steady breath.

6. Engage your back muscles to lift your chest and thighs higher, creating a bow shape with your body.

7. Hold this position for as long as is comfortable, continuing to breathe evenly.

8. To release, exhale and gently lower your chest, thighs, and feet back to the ground.

9. Rest with your head turned to one side and your arms alongside your body.

Drishti: Forward or towards the nose.

Contradictions:

• Flex the body as per your strength and ability. Overstretch can cause you harm, so don't overstretch your body.

• Don't get out of the asana in a rush. Gently release it. Besides, don't do it in a hurry. Conduct this steadily and smoothly.

• If you experience any type of muscle cramp or discomfort while doing this asana, release the asana immediately.

• If your muscles are tight or you are not flexible enough, try some simple yoga asana stretching at first before doing this asana.

• Avoid this asana in any recent or severe injury to the shoulder, back, arms, legs, core, and hips. Doing this asana in certain circumstances will bring you discomfort.

• When coping with physical disorders such as carpal tunnel syndrome, elevated or low blood pressure, hernia, spinal inflammation, or cardiac attacks, do not practice this asana.

Timing: 20-60 seconds

8. Paschimottanasana (Seated Forward Bend)

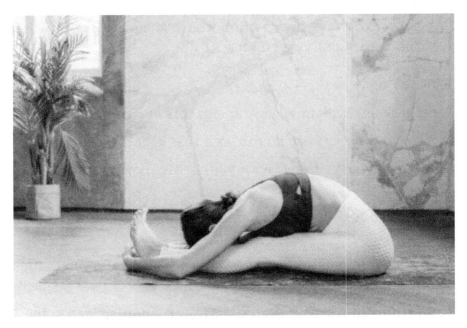

Paschimottanasana or Seated Forward Bend pumps a fresh volume of blood to your head. This allows the production of additional nutrients and fresh oxygen in the head, which eliminates discomfort immediately. This asana also works on the digestive tract. And if the headache is connected to the stomach, you will instantly feel relief.

Benefits:

• It calms the brain, which relieves stress and mild depression.

• It stretches the spine, the shoulders, and the hamstrings.

• It stimulates the liver, kidney, ovary, and uterus.

• It boosts digestive fire.

• It helps to relieve signs of menopause and menstrual discomfort.

• It relieves headaches and anxiety and decreases exhaustion.

• It is like a therapy for increased blood pressure, infertility, insomnia, and sinusitis.

• Ancient texts state that Paschimottanasana increases appetite, reduces obesity, and cures diseases.

How to Do:

1. Sit back on the floor with your legs spread out in front of you.

2. Keep your back straight with your toes bent towards you.

3. Breathe in as you raise both your arms above your head and stretch out.

4. Breathe out when you lean over and extend your torso over your legs, holding your spine erect.

5. You can rest your head just beyond your knees and your hands on the floor or interlock them at your feet.

6. Breathing in, lift your head slightly and lengthen your spine.

7. Breathing out, bring your navel to your knees.

8. Stay in this spot for 10-30 seconds.

9. Breathe in and get up while you raise your arms above your head.

10. Breathe out and bring your hands down.

11. Relax and try to feel the sensations in your body and mind.

Drishti: At the nose.

Contradictions:

• If you have an injury to your arms, hips, ankles, or shoulders, avoid this pose. Also, don't force yourself. If you're too tight to get a deep bend, just do what you can with no pain.

• Because this pose compresses the abdomen, it may not be comfortable with a full stomach.

Timing: 10-30 seconds

9. Kumbhakasana (High Plank)

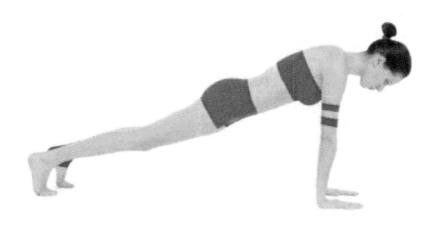

Plank is a purely fundamental pose. Being a part of the Sun Salutation sequence, it is also performed several times in the Ashtanga, Vinyasa, and Power Yoga classes. It teaches you to hold together—giving you the strength you need for dynamic poses, and the flexibility to float effortlessly through transitions between poses. A plank functions more than just the core, it develops abdominal strength; you may even shake while you practice it.

In a plank, you strengthen your arms, core muscles, butt, and front of your legs. When you perform this pose, your upper back and neck alignment will improve with time, and you will create support for your lower back while you continue to work your abdominals. However, it is necessary to work towards the formation of a well-aligned Plank Pose to achieve these benefits.

Benefits:

• Plank Pose exercises all the body's core muscles, including the belly, chest, and lower back.

• It helps you bring stability and strength on an emotional and spiritual level.

• It strengthens the arms, wrists, and shoulders and is also intended to brace the body for more challenging arm balances.

• Plank also activates the muscles around the spine, which improves posture.

• Practicing Plank Pose for a few minutes develops flexibility and stamina while toning the nervous system.

How to Do:

1. Begin on your four limbs, with your wrists under your shoulders and wrist creases parallel to the front edge of your mat.

2. Step one leg straight back, grounding all the toes. Next, step the other leg back.

3. Reach your heels back and firm your legs. Lift your kneecaps and press the tops of your thighs. Reach your tailbone back.

4. Push your hands and all your fingers steadily and evenly onto the mat and straighten the arms.

5. Hold for several minutes.

Drishti: Set your drishti at the tip of the nose.

Contradictions:

• Plank Pose should not be performed if one is injured in the arms or wrists, legs, or the upper leg at the thighs.

• Anybody struggling with low or high blood pressure should avoid this pose as a lot of pressure is experienced in the chest when balancing in the pose.

• Plank Pose can also be avoided by those with osteoporosis due to the possibility of fractures.

Timing: 1-3 minutes

10. Urdhva Mukha Svanasana (Upward-Facing Dog)

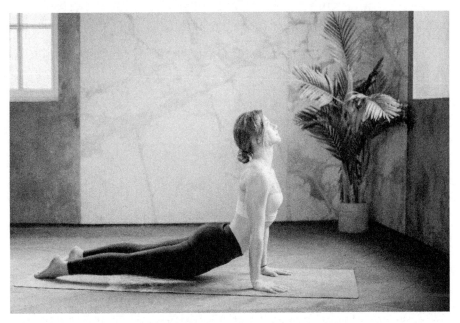

Upward-Facing Dog (Urdhva Mukha Svanasana) is a strong pose that awakens the energy of the upper body and offers a lovely stretch for the chest and abdomen while strengthening the wrists, arms, and shoulders.

Through strengthening and opening the upper body and chest, it strengthens body posture and can be beneficial for asthma. Upward Dog produces suppleness in the back torso and belly that strengthens the abdominal organs and improves digestion. They even firm the buttocks and thighs, helping to relieve sciatica. The backbend energizes and rejuvenates the body, offering relief from tiredness and mild depression.

Benefits:

• This powerful backbend helps to stretch the abdominals, chest, lungs, and shoulders while strengthening the arms and the posterior chain of the body, including the spinal erectors that help sustain good posture.

• It aims to maintain good posture and correct alignment.

• Correct alignment and good posture will contribute to reducing the occurrence of low back pain.

• Helps counteract regular forward flexion practices such as sitting, texting, or moving.

• Strengthens the spine, arms, and wrists.

• Firms the buttocks.

• Stimulates abdominal organs.

• Helps to relieve fatigue, mild depression, exhaustion, and sciatica.

• Beneficial for asthma.

How to Do:

1. Exhale as you gradually lower to the ground from Plank Pose. As your body approaches the ground, inhale and straighten your arms as you roll over your toes, switch your foot position from the toes tucked under to rest on the tops of your feet. If you can't turn off your toes, it's all right to move them one at a time. If you want, don't bring your thighs to the floor during the transition.

2. Open your chest towards the ceiling as you straighten your arms. Your gaze is going to rise slightly, but you need not throw your head back.

3. Hold your legs engaged and raise your hips from the floor. The only things that touch the floor are the palms of your hands and the tops of your feet.

4. Hold your shoulders above your wrists and draw your shoulder blades down and towards your spine to build room between your shoulders and ears.

5. Exhale and roll back over your toes to position the heels before you lift your hips to the Downward-Facing Dog.

Drishti: Nasagre Drishti (at the tip of the nose).

Contradictions:

• Avoid if you have any wrist, shoulder, or lower back injury, or ask any therapist how to adjust the pose if you decide to do so.

• To help avoid pain in the shoulders and wrists, make sure the alignment is right.

• Avoid this pose during the first trimester of pregnancy, and if you have a condition such as Carpal Tunnel that weakens the wrists.

Timing: 1-3 minutes

11. Adho Mukha Svanasana (Downward-Facing Dog)

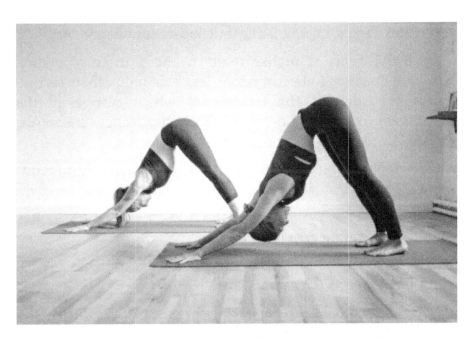

Among the most recognized yoga poses in the West, Downward-Facing Dog is a standing pose and a gentle inversion that builds strength while relaxing the entire body. It's called for the way dogs spontaneously extend their entire body! Downward-Facing Dog (sometimes referred to as 'Downward Dog' or 'Down Dog') is an integral part of Sun Salutation, which is sometimes practiced several times during a yoga session. This may be seen as a transitional posture, a resting stance, and a strength-builder.

This move lets you stretch your calves, hamstrings, and feet, open your shoulders and get the blood circulating into your body. It's a reboot to connect a little more to the core.

Benefits:

• Downward-Facing Dog energizes and rejuvenates the entire body.

• It flexes your hamstrings, shoulders, calves, arches, hands, and back deeply while building strength in your arms, shoulders, and legs.

• It creates a sense of well-being and boosts confidence.

• Since the heart is higher than the head in this posture, it is called a moderate inversion (less strenuous than certain inversions, such as the Headstand) which carries all the advantages of inversion—relief from headaches, insomnia, exhaustion, and slight depression.

• The supply of blood to the brain also soothes the nervous system, increases memory and concentration, and relieves stress.

• It can relieve anxiety and depression.

• Daily practice of this pose can boost digestion, ease back pain, and help prevent osteoporosis.

• It is also considered beneficial for sinusitis, asthma, flat feet, and signs of menopause.

How to Do:

1. Come onto your hands and knees with your wrists under your shoulders and your knees under your hips.

2. Curl your toes under and push back through your hands to raise your hips and straighten your legs.

3. Open your fingers and ground down from your forearms to your fingertips.

4. Shift the upper arms outward to extend the collarbones.

5. Let your head hang and push your shoulder blades away from your ears to your hips.

6. Engage the quadriceps to keep the weight of your body off your arms. Such a gesture goes a fair way towards rendering this a resting posture.

7. Rotate your thighs inward, keep your butt high, and lower your heels to the floor.

8. Check that the distance between your hands and feet is correct by moving forward to the position of the plank. For these two poses, the distance between the hands and the feet should be the same. Do not step your feet towards the hands in Down Dog to bring the heels to the floor.

9. Hold for 5 breaths or more, as per your will. Exhale and bend your knees to let go and come back to your hands and knees.

Drishti: Nasagre Drishti (focus at the tip of your nose).

Contradictions:

• If you have Carpal Tunnel Syndrome or other wrist disorders, this pose is not suggested.

• People with back injuries, arms, or legs should also avoid this.

• People with elevated blood pressure and eye or inner ear

disorders should also avoid it.

Timing: 1 minute

12. Utthita Parsvakonasana (Side Angle Pose)

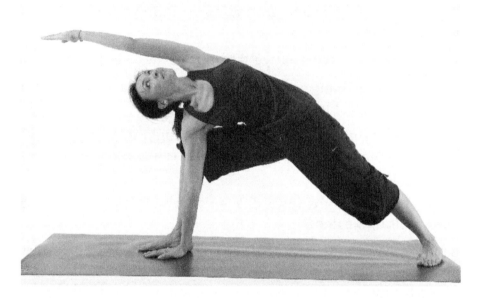

Revolved Side Angle Pose is a deep, standing twist that challenges the balance and strengthens the legs and core. It's a powerful variation of the Extended Side Angle Pose (Utthita Parsvakonasana). It also combines the benefits of Warrior I (Virabhadrasana I) and Crescent Lunge Twist (Parivrtta Anjaneyasana).

Benefits:

• One of the greatest advantages of a side stretch for a spiritual seeker is that the nerves on both sides of the spinal cord are effectively flexed. As a result, the flow of prana energy becomes smooth and correct.

• The Revolved Side Angle stretches, tones, and strengthens the entire body, inside and out.

• It stretches the thighs, knees, ankles, calves, groins, chest, and shoulders.

• Helps to balance your mind, even in stressful situations.

• This pose builds strength in the legs and, in particular, in the quadriceps and ankles.

• It also strengthens and tones the abdominal organs and lungs, which improves digestion, elimination, metabolism, and breathability.

• This pose challenges and enhances balance, and helps to develop stamina and full-body coordination.

• It boosts focus and improves strength and confidence.

• It relieves stiffness in the shoulders which may even be helpful for low back pain and sciatica.

• In fact, twisting detoxifies the body by promoting fresh blood flow through the organs, particularly the kidneys, liver, and spleen.

• This intense twist will help wring out contaminants that hinder the body from functioning at its best!

How to Do:

1. From Downward-Facing Dog, bring your right foot forward to the inside of your right hand. The toes are meant to be in contact with the fingers.

2. Bend your right knee and give your calf and thigh a right angle with the thigh parallel to the floor.

3. Pivot on the ball of your left foot to bring your left heel down to the floor.

4. Flatten your left hand to the floor under your left shoulder.

5. Drag your belly button towards your spine while you raise

your torso to your right knee, open your chest, and stack your left shoulder on top of your right.

6. Point your left arm forward as shown in the figure. Bring your gaze to your left hand.

7. Stay in for several breaths. Step back to the Downward Dog and repeat the pose with your left foot forward.

Drishti: Hastagrai Drishti (towards the hand).

Contradictions:

• You should avoid this pose if you have a neck, back, or shoulder injury.

• Because it needs balance, it is not advised if you have high or low blood pressure or if you are pregnant.

• If you have an injury of the hip, back, shoulder, or knee, speak to a doctor or yoga trainer and see if it is appropriate to perform this pose or not.

• If you have diarrhea, avoid this pose.

Timing: 30-60 seconds, on each leg

13. Utthita Trikonasana (Triangle Pose)

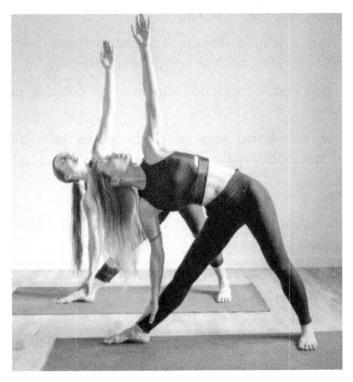

Trikonasana, or Triangle Pose, is performed next in the sequence to revitalize, reinforce, and stretch the mind and body. The hips, the legs, and the core will be the focus of this pose.

Benefits:

• Triangle Pose is a deep stretch for the hamstrings, groins, and hips; Trikonasana also opens the chest and shoulders.

• Healthy release and understanding of our emotions are key to living a balanced life, and practicing Triangle Pose is a tremendously powerful way to open the hips physically and energetically.

• It significantly reduces back pain, stress, and slow digestion.

• This pose strengthens the muscles of the thighs, hips, and back while toning the knees and ankles.

• It is considered to be good for anxiety, flat feet, infertility, osteoporosis, and even sciatica.

• More than a simple stretch, Trikonasana improves overall balance and stability, both physically and mentally.

• It increases body confidence and courage, creating poise and grace both on and off the mat.

• It has a wonderful way of aligning yourself—physically, mentally, and emotionally.

How to Do:

1. Start by standing in Utthita Tadasana (Five-Pointed Star Pose), and take a few breaths.

2. From here, turn your right foot outwards to 90°.

3. Inhale and stretch the torso to the right side, bending gradually at the hips.

4. Exhale, bring the right hand to the floor, and place it behind your right foot. Next, inhale and stretch your left arm up and, as you exhale, look up at the raised arm.

5. Inhale and keep the body loose to adjust the hips and feet and make sure the alignment is perfect to make the body comfortable.

6. Exhale and move deeper into the pose. Stay in Trikonasana (Triangle Pose) for 6 breaths or more, breathing and extending the arms and torso deeper.

7. Inhale, loosen the torso and relax in Utthita Tadasana. Relax and repeat, taking the torso to the left while extending the right arm up.

8. Stay on the left side for 6 breaths or more as well.

9. Release and relax.

Drishti: Hastagrai Drishti (gazing at the hand) or towards the ceiling.

Contradictions:

• Avoid doing this pose if you are suffering from migraine, diarrhea, low or high blood pressure, or neck and back injuries.

• Those with high blood pressure may do this pose but without raising their hand overhead, as this may further raise the blood pressure.

Timing: 20-60 seconds, on each side

14. Uttanasana (Standing Forward Bend)

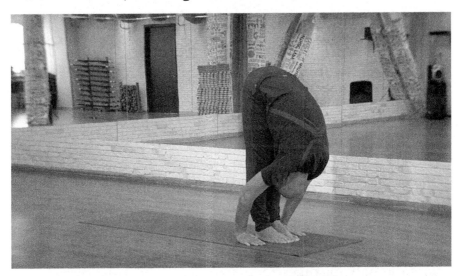

The back of the body is where all the major muscles are. Standing Forward Bend loosens up and activates the back body. These muscles play a significant role in strengthening the spine and linking the legs to the upper body. We gain trust and coordination by reinforcing the back body. When we understand the body better, we can move out of our comfort zone and practice deeper. Through daily practice, we achieve consistency and recognize that there are obstacles to propel us toward our target.

The end pose leaves you in such a position that your head is in the lower stratum with your heart. This enables a splash of blood to the head, and a revamping of the blood cells, leaving you with a sense of novelty. This posture is also strongly recommended for individuals who are dealing with asthma or mild depression.

Benefits:

· Calms the brain and helps ease stress and mild depression.

· Stimulates the liver and kidneys.

· Strengthens the thighs and knees.

· Improves digestion.

· Aims to ease the effects of menopause.

· Decreases exhaustion and anxiety.

· Relieves headaches and insomnia.

· This asana offers you a healthy stretch for your back, hips, calves, and hamstrings.

· It calms your mind and relieves your anxiety. It also holds the mind calm.

· It helps to alleviate headaches and insomnia.

· This bend provides a pleasant massage to the digestive organs, thereby enhancing digestion.

· Menopause and menstrual problems are eased.

· This asana aims to cure elevated blood pressure, asthma, infertility, sinusitis, and osteoporosis.

How to Do:

1. From Raised Hands Pose (Urdhva Hastasana) with arms stretching overhead, sweep your arms down each side of your body to a forward fold from your hips. This is also referred to as

a Swan Dive.

2. Bring your fingers in line with your toes. If you can, press your palms flat on the mat. If they don't reach the floor, you can use blocks under your hands.

3. Bend the knees a bit so they won't be locked.

4. Engage and draw the quadriceps muscles. The more you use your quads, the more the hamstrings (the muscles on the back of the thighs) open up.

5. Bring your weight a little forward onto the balls of your feet and hold your hips over your ankles.

6. Permit your head to hang.

7. To come up, inhale and put your hands on your hips. Push down your tailbone and flex your stomach muscles as you steadily rise.

Drishti: Focus your eyes on a fixed point in front of you.

Contradictions:

• If you have the following issues, skip this asana:

- Lower back injury
- A tear in the hamstring
- Sciatica
- Glaucoma or retinal detachment

• If you have a back injury, do this asana keeping your knees bent. You may also do the Ardha Uttanasana by putting your hands on a wall, such that they're parallel to the floor. Make sure that your legs are perpendicular to your torso.

• Women who are pregnant or menstruating should not bend over fully. Do Ardha Uttanasana by holding the spine parallel to the floor and the palms on the wall, holding the abdomen soft and the back straight.

• Those with spinal herniation should not lean over fully, and they should do this asana with a concave back with their palms on the blocks.

Timing: 20-60 seconds

15. Tadasana (Mountain Pose)

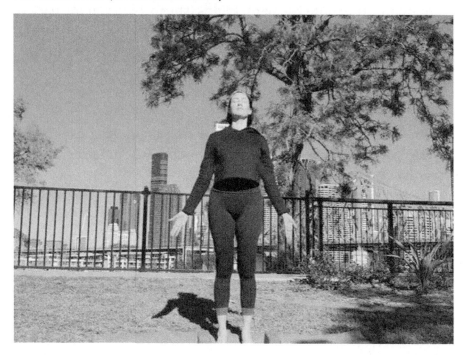

Also known as Samsthithi, or Equal Standing, this pose is essentially the simple act of standing up straight with an upright and alert posture, but like so many things in yoga, the details are limitless, and the simplest things are often the hardest to master.

The alignment that you learn in Tadasana will translate into almost every other pose in practice. Sometimes in subtle ways, but often in self-explanatory ones.

Tadasana shows one how to activate every muscle group in the body and how to articulate every joint complex to create a pose that enables energy and knowledge to flow freely around the body. Mountain Pose cultivates many spiritual benefits as well, in particular prana, the life force of the body.

Benefits:

• Tadasana unites the Crown Chakra, the Brow Chakra, the Heart Chakra, and the Navel Chakra to provide you with mental and physical benefits.

• Tadasana helps relieve anxiety by focusing further on breath control.

• It also helps to encourage the body to work more effortlessly as you develop a more stable and grounded practice.

• Combat fatigue.

• Soothes the mind (stress, depression).

• Stimulates the circulation of blood.

• Brings oxygen to the upper body and the brain.

• Assists in bone growth (makes you taller).

• Reinforces the back nerves.

• Stretches your back, arms, and legs.

• Boosts digestion.

• Stops osteoporosis.

• Tadasana helps us confront our subtle, energetic body.

• Tadasana shows one how to add meditation to daily life.

How to Do:

1. Standing firm pick up all the toes and fan them out, then lower them back down to build a proper, stable foundation. You can separate your heels somewhat if your knees get uncomfortable.

2. Let the legs and calves be rooted down to the floor.

3. Engage the quadriceps (the muscles at the front of the thighs) and pull them forward, allowing your kneecaps to rise.

4. Rotate the thighs backward, producing a widening of the sit bones.

5. Hold the spine's natural curves in position.

6. Tone your belly, drawing it in slightly.

7. Widen your collarbones and ensure that your shoulders are on your pelvis.

8. Shrug your shoulders to your ears and roll them back to release your shoulder blades to your back.

9. Let your arms hang naturally with your elbows slightly bent with your palms facing forward.

10. Your neck is long, your jaw is neither tucked up nor raised, and the crown of your head rises to the ceiling.

11. Once you've checked all of your alignment points, take at least 5-10 long breaths while you're in this pose.

Drishti: Drishti may vary, but a forward, neutral, soft gaze is common.

Contradiction:

• Owing to the balancing aspect of your posture, you should not perform Mountain Pose if you're experiencing headaches, insomnia, low blood pressure, or if you are lightheaded and/or dizzy.

• Always operate within your own set of limitations and skills. Talk to the doctor before doing yoga if you have any medical issues.

Timing: 1-3 minutes

16. Utthita Hasta Padangustasana (Extended Hand-To-Big-Toe Pose)

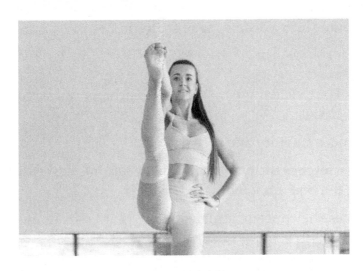

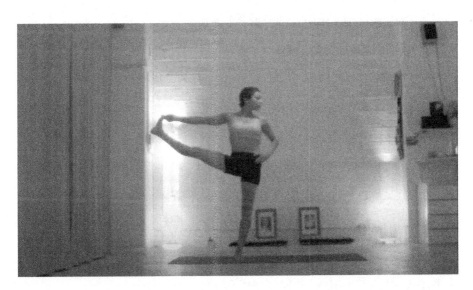

Utthita Hasta Padangusthasana, also known as the Extended Hand-To-Toe Pose, is a challenging and invigorating posture that stretches and strengthens while calming the mind and improving focus.

When we balance on one leg in this pose, with the body held tall, the front and back of the body equally open, with awareness spreading through all the cells, our whole being enters a state of balance. Our energy, nerve flow, mind, body, and breath unite and we enter into a deep state of stillness.

Benefits:

• Utthita Hasta Padangusthasana strengthens and stretches the legs and ankles.

• It enhances stability and focus.

• Deeply stretches the hamstrings (back leg muscles) while softly opening the hips, shoulders, and arms.

• Enhances the concentrating capacity that helps in meditation practices.

• This strengthens the Svadhishthana Chakra (Sacral Chakra).

• It lengthens the spine from the base.

• This helps in relieving anxiety.

• It strengthens the nervous system.

• Your physical body gets revitalized.

• It improves the flexibility of the hips.

• It opens the chest and the shoulders.

• It activates the joints.

• It reduces symptoms of rheumatic disorder.

How to Do:

1. Begin in Tadasana/Mountain Pose.

2. Take a point at your eye level to focus with a soft gaze.

3. As you exhale, shift your weight to your left foot and lift your right knee. Reach the big toe with your right hand.

4. Firm your left hip and lengthen your spine. Hold your shoulder blades firmly on your back with your chest open. As you inhale, start extending your right leg to the front, without losing the length of the spine.

5. Stay for 5 breaths or longer, then as you inhale, take your leg out to the right and stay for 5 or more breaths.

6. Bring your leg back to the center to get out of the pose, on an inhalation. As you exhale, drop your foot back to the floor.

7. Repeat on the other side.

Drishti: At a fixed point ahead.

Contradictions:

• If you have a recent or chronic ankle or low back injury, do not perform this pose.

• Though this pose is good for increasing blood circulation in the legs and providing a toned look to the entire leg, hamstring, quadriceps, and calves, an injury will only do further damage. It is best to take precautions before performing this pose, even with a hip injury.

• Pregnant women should always be cautious of their balance in this pose and consider using a chair or wall for support.

Timing: 20-60 seconds

17. Sirsasana (Headstand)

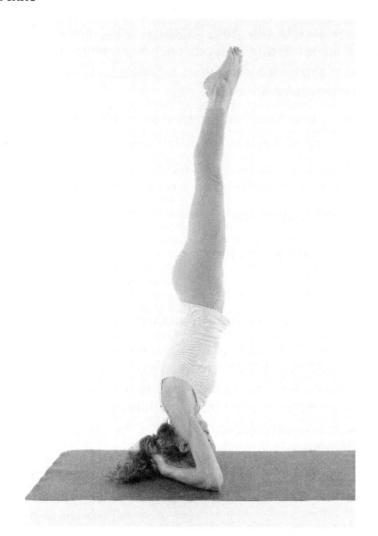

Headstand is pointed to as the 'King of Asanas' because of its significant benefits to the body and mind. When you do a Headstand, not only does the body invert but also the blood pressure. Pressure changes in the head, neck, shoulders, veins, arteries, lungs, and legs. This change in blood pressure causes the body to adapt to retain equilibrium in the various processes of the body. The upper limb muscles and tissues are often strained and stimulated.

The Headstand raises the overall prana, and it also converts sexual energy into spiritual energy, known as 'Ojas.' Increased Ojas will enhance spiritual practices, such as meditation. Headstand also provides a whole different way to look at the universe by flipping you upside down.

Benefits:

• Enhances the activity of the pineal, hypothalamus, and pituitary glands. This aims to enhance the functioning and coordination of all endocrine glands.

• Enhances the capacity of the body to sustain homeostasis by activating the nervous system.

• Delivers conditioning to the head, eyes, and ears due to elevated blood pressure.

• Enhanced memory and concentration.

• Reduction of emotional stress, depression, and anxiety.

• Improves the activity of the Central Nervous System.

• Enhances the body's capacity to monitor blood pressure by activating so-called baroreceptors.

• Provides rest to the heart by reversing the blood pressure.

• Strengthens body posture and triggers the core.

• Improves memory.

• Trains body and mind for meditation

• Improves self-control and sexual sublimation.

• Is extremely effective when practiced while chanting the mantra and regulating the breath.

• Brightens psychic faculties

• Support us to gain a new perspective.

• Reinforces the muscles of the spine, shoulders, and arms.

• Enhances blood and lymph supply in the body.

• Improves digestion and elimination.

How to Do:

1. Sit down on your knees and raise your elbows to measure the optimal distance. Then drop your arms to the ground under your shoulders.

2. Keep your elbows there, bring your hands together and interlock your fingers such that your arms form a triangle. Don't let your elbows open.

3. Place your head on the ground with the back of your head in your cupped hands.

4. Curl your toes, bend your knees, and push your hips to the sky.

5. Bring the right knee to the chest and add the other knee. That'll make your back straight.

6. As you inhale, push your legs to the sky. Bring your focus to a steady point, ideally at eye level. Take easy relaxing breaths and keep the pose as long as possible.

Drishti: Forward, at a fixed point.

Contradictions:

• Infants under the age of 7 years are not allowed to do this as their skull is newly fused and could also be soft and susceptible to injury.

• Pregnant women should avoid it as it could be dangerous if they slip out of their pose for some reason.

• If you have glaucoma, avoid it as it can raise the pressure in your eyes.

• If you have an acute headache or serious migraine, the Headstand should be avoided.

• Persons with shoulder and neck injuries should also avoid

it until the damage is healed.

• People with hypertension should avoid Headstand and all inversions.

• People with serious heart problems should avoid it.

• People suffering from osteoporosis should also avoid Headstand.

Timing: 10-60 seconds

18. Vriksasana (Tree Pose)

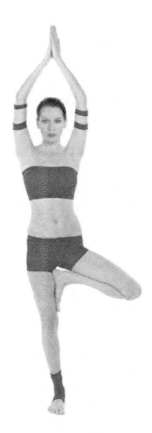

Vriksasana is one of the basic standing asanas and is considered an important balancing posture. It teaches us to reclaim our center, helps us feel fully supported on one leg, improves concentration, and cultivates grace and ease of body and mind.

If you've ever tripped off a curb or fallen on a patch of ice, you're sure to appreciate the value of having a moral sense of balance. Practicing balancing poses in yoga, such as Tree Pose, can help you achieve physical and mental stability and well-being.

The labyrinthine branches and roots of the real tree echo the nervous and circulatory systems of the human body. We refer to the bronchial as 'branches' of our lungs, arteries, and nerves. Our spine, like the trunk of a tree, is the foundation of our well-being.

The advantages of Vriksasana are strengthened as the yogi sees these parallels between the tree, the human body, and the psyche. Visualizing energy from roots (feet), branches (arms and fingers), and crown (head), then spiraling through the chakras (energy centers in the body) up the trunk (spin) is sure to trigger Kundalini Shakti.

Benefits:

• It provides harmony and balance to the mind.

• It helps to boost focus.

• It extends the entire body from the knees to the fingers, rejuvenating you.

• It brings peace of mind; good for those who are facing the dilemma of depression and anxiety.

• It enhances endurance, concentration, and immunity.

• It's good for the hips since it makes you open them up.

• It's helpful for people who have sciatica.

• It increases the flexibility of muscles of the legs, back, and chest.

• It makes the ankles stronger.

• The person who has trouble with the knee must perform this.

• Strengthens thighs and calves.

• It is effective in improving memory, attention, and other cognitive ability of the mind and mental well-being.

• It stabilizes the nervous system and soothes the mind by relieving fear and tension.

• Brings the greatest natural coordination of neuromuscular action.

• It provides the necessary stretching to the groins.

• The person suffering from a flat foot should practice it.

• It makes you more focused and concentrated.

• While doing this asana, the ligaments and tendons of the legs are strengthened.

• It's healthy for the pelvic area, too.

• It builds self-esteem and self-confidence.

• It calms down and relaxes the central nervous system.

• It helps ease rheumatic pain and even treats numbness.

• Vriksasana calms your mind and makes your body steady and solid.

How to Do:

1. From a standing position, raise the right heel to the crotch. Press the heel of the foot into the inner thigh, with the toes facing the floor. Make sure the left leg is straight. Find harmony.

2. When you are well positioned, take a deep breath, gracefully lift your arms from the side above your head and bring your palms together in the 'Namaste' Mudra (hands-folded position).

3. Set the shoulders down, raise the chest, and pull the chin to the neck lock. See straight ahead in front of you, at a distant

object. A focused gaze helps to maintain a steady equilibrium.

4. Make sure that your back is straight. Your whole body should be as taut as a stretched elastic band. Start taking slow, deep breaths. Relax the body more and more with each exhalation. Just be in your body and breathe with a gentle smile on your face.

5. Use Mula Bandha to secure the pelvis beneath. Don't stick your buttocks out.

6. Stay here for 1-5 minutes, depending on your ability. To exit, gently put your hands down from the sides with a gradual exhalation. You should release the right leg gently.

7. Stand erect and upright as you did at the beginning of your pose. Repeat this pose with your left leg off the ground on your right thigh.

Drishti: In Vriksasana, anchoring your gaze on the horizon or a fixed point directs energy forward to keep you upright.

Contradictions:

· Due to the balancing aspect of your posture, do not exercise Tree Pose if you are already having headaches, insomnia, low blood pressure, or if you feel lightheaded and/or dizzy.

· Those with elevated blood pressure should not raise their arms overhead; instead join them in front of your chest.

Timing: 20-60 seconds, on each leg

19. Prasarita Padottanasana (Wide-Legged Forward Fold)

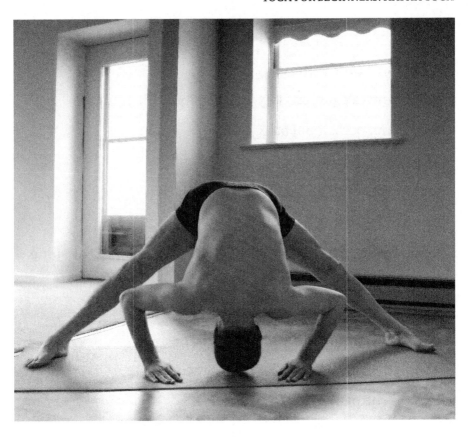

Wide-Legged Forward Bend (or Prasarita Padottanasana) is an energizing inversion that improves circulation to the brain while giving a deep stretch to the legs, back, and arms. The pose gets its name from Sanskrit terms, 'Prasarita,' meaning outstretched, 'Pada,' meaning foot, 'Ut,' meaning intense, 'Tan,' meaning spread or stretch, and 'Asana,' meaning pose.

Practicing Prasarita Padottanasana every day can be intense, spacious, and soothing after a long period of standing poses, or mostly after some physical exercise, such as running, walking, or cycling. More frequently than not, this asana is sequenced toward the end of the yoga session. It's a good preparatory yoga pose for a Headstand and Peacock Pose. Once this pose is mastered, you can always go for several other variations of this pose for higher results.

Benefits:

• Results in a calmer mind.

• Relief from fatigue, anxiety, and moderate depression.

• Relief from occasional back pain.

• Helps open hips.

• Relief from strain in the neck and shoulder.

• Improved digestion.

• Supports and stretches the inner and back legs and the spine.

• Tones the abdominal organs.

• Eases the brain.

• Stretch the back and the inside of the legs.

• Stretch the back, shoulders, and chest.

• Relieves the pain in the upper back.

How to Do:

1. Step your legs 3-4 feet apart from Mountain Pose into Five-Pointed Star Pose. With a flat back, exhale and drop the palms to the floor under the shoulders.

2. Use your arms to bring your forehead down to the surface, leaning your knees to the back wall. Press onto the feet, and lengthen the legs to press the hips towards the ceiling.

3. Feel the spine pulled in opposite directions as you press your head down and raise your hips.

4. Breathe and hang on for 3-10 breaths.

5. To release, reach out to the sides with your arms and inhale back towards the Five-Pointed Star.

Drishti: Focus your gaze inward (on your Third Eye/between your brows).

Contradictions:

• Persons with lower back problems should not practice this asana.

• Individuals who have concerns with their knees are also not recommended to perform this asana.

Timing: 20-60 seconds

20. Virabhadrasana I (Warrior I)

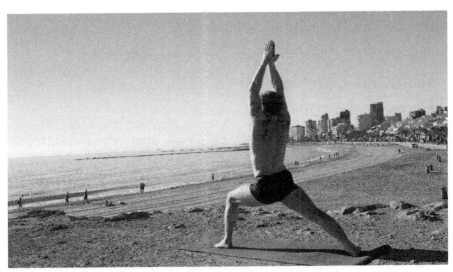

Who was Virabhadra, the one that these Warrior Poses are named after? He was Lord Shiva, the Hindu god who reflects destruction (or dissolution of the world back into the Holy Spirit) and a great protector of the sages.

Virabhadra (which means "Distinguished Hero") was one of the attendants of Lord Shiva who slayed several demons and performed various good deeds to defend holy beings in Hindu mythology. Some people consider him an incarnation of Lord

Shiva himself.

What's being commemorated in this pose's name, and held up as an ideal for all practitioners, is the "Spiritual Warrior," who bravely does battle with the universal enemy, self-ignorance (Avidya), the ultimate source of all our suffering.

So when we perform any of the Virabhadrasana, we strive to reflect the inner attributes of one of the most admired embodiments of the warrior archetype. These fighter qualities are empowerment, courage, clarity, and lack of attachment.

This pose strengthens the arms, shoulders, thighs, and back muscles, all in one go.

Benefits:

• Stretches the chest, lungs, shoulders, neck, stomach, and groin.

• Supports the back of the shoulders, arms, and muscles.

• Strengthens and extends thighs, calves, and ankles.

• Therapeutic for Sciatica.

• By opening the chest, Warrior I can open your heart and develop your courage.

• It lets you develop inner strength and bravery while helping you to open up to yourself and others.

• Energizes the entire body.

• The physical, mental, and emotional benefits of Warrior I lead to balanced well-being and to the physical, mental, and spiritual connection that yoga offers.

How to Do:

1. From the Mountain Pose, take a big step back with your left leg, such that your left foot is about 45° to the left. The body faces the front of the mat.

2. Bend the left knee and thigh, holding the weight in the front heel and the big toe and the right foot should be pressing from the outer heel.

3. Square your hips to make sure your knee is directly over your ankle. Upon inhalation, raise your arms straight, releasing your shoulders from the ears, and spread your shoulder blades.

4. Join both your hands over the head in Namaste Mudra. Hang in the pose for 10-15 breaths.

5. Get out of the pose with an inhalation, press your right heel as you straighten your left leg and lower the arms. Move back to the Mountain Pose before you perform the pose on the other side.

Drishti: Urdhva Drishti, gazing up to infinity.

Contradictions:

• High blood pressure and heart patients should avoid it.

Timing: 20-60 seconds, on each side

21. Virabhadrasana II (Warrior II)

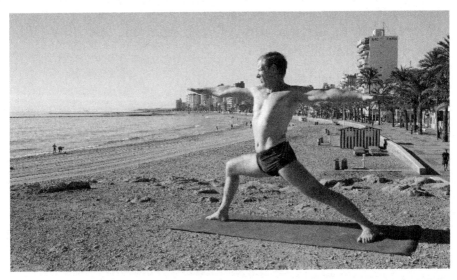

Virabhadrasana II (Warrior Pose II) is then 2nd in the sequence of 3 yoga poses that carry out the noble qualities that exist in each of us. This Virabhadrasana builds strength and stamina. This Warrior Pose improves and tones the muscles of the calf, the quadriceps, and the buttocks. It opens the hips and shoulders, tones the arms, extends the chest, improves the lung capacity, and stretches the muscles of the chest. The stomach muscles and organs are toned down to aid digestion. The circulation and transfer of energy across the body are also improved.

Benefits:

· Supports and stretches the legs and ankles.

· Develops harmony and equilibrium.

· Stretches the groins, the chest, the lungs, and the shoulders.

· Activates abdominal organs.

· Increases stamina.

· Relieves back pain, particularly during the 2nd trimester of pregnancy.

· Therapeutic to Carpal Tunnel Syndrome, flat feet, infertility, osteoporosis, and sciatica.

· Activates the Navel/Solar Plexus Chakra.

· Offers a mentality of a warrior, increases determination, willpower, and endurance.

How to Do:

1. Turn the right toe to the right from Five-Pointed Star and bend the right knee directly over the right ankle.

2. Turn the hips and shoulders towards the front and stretch out through the fingertips.

3. Look at the middle right finger, pressing on your feet and holding your legs strong.

4. Sink the hips to the surface, then meet the crown of the head to lengthen the spine. Relax your shoulders down and back, pressing your chest forward.

5. Breathe and hang on for several deep breaths.

6. To release, straighten the legs and bring them back to the Five-Pointed Star.

Drishti: Urdhva Drishti, gazing up or outward has an expansive feeling of gazing out towards infinity.

Contradictions:

• Those with medical issues that influence balance should not perform this.

• Stop practicing Virabhadrasana II in extreme knee pain, elevated blood pressure, or chronic neck or shoulder injuries.

• Stop turning your head when holding the asana if you're someone with a neck issue. Instead, keep staring straight ahead without straining the neck.

• Be patient while performing Virabhadrasana II if you have diarrhea.

Timing: 30-60 seconds, on each side

22. Virabhadrasana III (Warrior III)

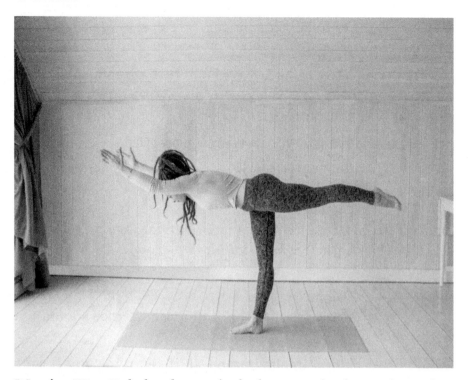

Warrior III or Tuladandasana is the last pose in the Hatha series. Once again requiring balance, determination, and core strength, this pose also increases circulation (especially in the heart and brain).

It's a pose that tests the body in both backward and forward bending components. It also develops strength and grounding in the legs, thus providing a chance for lightness and play. It could even open your eyes to new ways of practicing.

Benefits:

• Provides full relief of spinal stress.

• Increases cardiovascular circulation, particularly in the blood vessels of the heart.

• Refine control and balance by enhancing physical and mental powers.

• It brings your attention inward.

• Improves posture.

• Relieves the pain of the spine.

• Eliminates varicose veins.

• Exercises liver, pancreas, spleen, and circulatory and nervous systems.

• May help clear blocked arteries and prevent heart problems.

• Perfects control and co-ordination.

• Firms hips, buttocks, and upper thighs, and provides many of the same benefits for the legs as for Standing Head to Knee.

• Increases circulation and strengthens the cardiovascular system, which is an excellent exercise for poor posture.

• Improves the flexibility, strength, and muscle tone of the shoulders, upper arms, spine, and hip joints.

• Helps to relieve depression, memory loss, and constipation.

• Increases the function of the brain and adrenal glands.

• Builds a relation of power and harmony.

• Stretch the spine and back of the legs.

• It allows you to ignite your fire and live intentionally.

How to Do:

1. From Mountain Pose, move your right foot forward and transfer all your weight to this leg.

2. Inhale and raise your arms above your head, if you want you can interlace your thumbs, pointing up the index finger.

3. As you exhale, raise your left leg up and out, hinging your hips to lower your arms and torso down to the floor.

4. Reach out through the left toes and the crown and fingertips, forming a straight line.

5. Breathe and hang on for 2-20 breaths.

6. To release, inhale and bring your arms and leg down to the floor and shift both legs back to Mountain Pose.

7. Repeat on the other side.

Drishti: Focus on the Third Eye.

Contradictions:

• Anybody with high blood pressure should not do this asana, as the body needs to be focused to remain balanced. The sudden flow of blood to the brain may not be suited to practitioners suffering from blood pressure.

• Individuals suffering from back problems should avoid this or should do so on a step-by-step basis.

• Some find it difficult to look down and may suffer from migraine, which causes dizziness.

• Spondylitis is another case where practitioners should avoid this asana.

Timing: 30-60 seconds, on each side

Savasana (Corpse Pose)

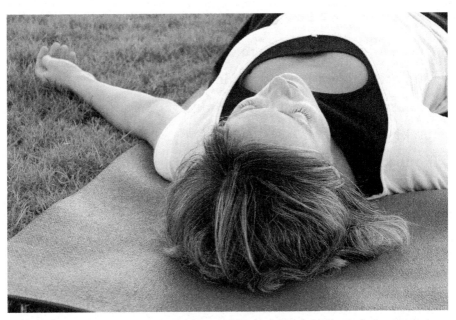

A good yoga session always ends in Savasana. The Savasana or the Corpse Pose is the ultimate climax to a great yoga session. It induces a deep state of rest in the body. The body almost drifts into a meditative trance and becomes rejuvenated. The rejuvenation also banishes migraines.

It's a wonderful opportunity to turn energies inward and rebuild and revitalize the hard-working mind and body. Expanding on the mental benefits, Savasana offers a chance to discover the 5th limb in yoga—Pratyahara. Quite simplistic, Pratyahara is withdrawing from the senses and gaining control over external influences.

However, the art of Pratyahara is very complex, leading to the fact that Savasana is one of the most challenging poses to master. Lying here for up to 5-10 minutes, based on how much time you've, lets you calm your entire body and mind before you get back to life.

Benefits:

• It brings your focus to the breath.

• It maximizes the release of stress by relaxing the entire body.

• It calms your heart's rhythm and reduces blood pressure.

• It reduces exhaustion and headaches.

• It relaxes the mind, reduces insomnia, and improves sleep.

• It relieves jet lag.

• It improves the absorption of nutrients.

• It improves blood pressure, brain waves, and respiratory rate.

• It strengthens the immune response.

• It optimizes the circulation of newly oxygenated blood through the body.

• It relaxes and focuses your mind.

• It brings the body to a normal state of balance, like blood pressure, heart rate, and brain waves.

• Helps you achieve complete relaxation of the physical body.

• Results in a calmer, positive mind.

• Improves focus and concentration.

• Reduced blood pressure.

• Raises awareness of the "Inner You."

• Helps you let go of the ego and attachment to material things.

• Establishes a connection with the spiritual source.

How to Do:

1. Lie back on the floor and rest your legs apart.

2. Relax your arms by softly allowing them to fall to both sides with the palms facing up.

3. Close your eyes now.

4. Ensure that the fingertips and toes are relaxed to eliminate

any limitations on the throat.

5. Pull the shoulders down and flat against the floor.

6. Choose a spot on the floor where the body is at ease.

7. Breathe gradually and intensely, enabling the body to eliminate more tension with each exhalation.

8. Focus on breathing, especially if your mind is wandering around.

Drishti: Nasagre Drishti (tip of the nose).

Contradictions:

• Savasana is appropriate for all yoga students, but still, if you're uncomfortable lying on your back, try a sponsored variation of the pose.

• Women who are pregnant should keep their head and chest raised by resting on a bolster or a cushion.

Timing: 5-10 minutes

Hatha Yoga Pranayamas

1. Nadi Shodhana (Alternate Nostril Breathing)

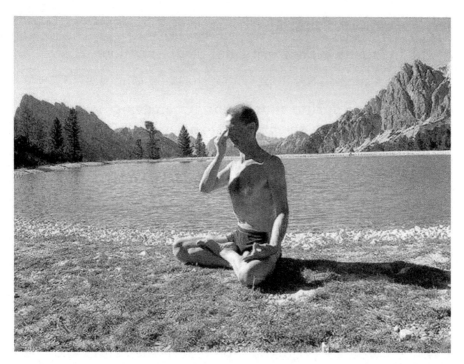

'Nadi' means a subtle energy channel and 'Shodhan' means cleaning and purification. Nadis are subtle energy pathways in the human body that can be blocked because of a variety of reasons. Alternative Nostril Breathing produces a calm, harmonious sensation that integrates the left and right hemispheres of the brain.

It is a relaxation practice that helps clear these blocked energy pathways and soothes the mind. The technique is also known as Anulom Vilom Pranayama.

Benefits:

• Nadi Shodhan Pranayama makes the mind calm and allows it to enter a meditative state.

• Practicing it for only a few minutes a day helps keep the mind relaxed, content, and quiet.

• It helps to relieve chronic anxiety and exhaustion.

• Excellent relaxation technique to relax the mind and center it.

• Our mind tends to regret or glorify the past and gets anxious about the future. Nadi Shodhan Pranayama helps bring the mind back to the present moment.

• Works therapeutically for the bulk of circulatory and respiratory disorders.

• Releases chronic tension in the body and mind rapidly and helps to calm.

• Helps to align the left and right hemispheres of the brain, which correspond to the cognitive and emotional dimensions of our personality.

• Helps to purify and align the nadis—the subtle energy pathways, providing a steady flow of prana in the body.

• Maintains the temperature of the body.

How to Do:

1. Sit back with a straight spine. You could be in Easy Pose or on a chair, anywhere you can keep your spine straight and relaxed. Your left hand will be in Gyan Mudra on your left knee.

Mudra and Breath: Use the thumb and index fingers of the right hand to make a "U" of the two fingers, use the thumb to close the right nostril and the index finger to close the left one.

2. Close your eyes and focus on your Third Eye. Breathe calmly, heavily, and full, as you perform the following sequence:

- Inhale through the left nostril, closing the right nostril with the right thumb.
- Exhale through your right nostril, closing your left nostril with the index finger.
- Inhale through your right nostril, closing your left nostril with the index finger.
- Exhale through your left nostril, closing your right nostril with your thumb.

7. To end, inhale deeply, hold your breath for a few seconds, lower your hand, and exhale.

Drishti: Focus on your Third Eye.

Contradictions:

• This practice is better avoided for those suffering from hypertension.

• Not to be performed in the full stomach, since this may contribute to digestive issues that further put a strain on internal organs such as the stomach.

• It is best to take the advice of a yoga practitioner if suffering from migraines. A wrong practice could aggravate the problems.

Timing: 3-5 minutes

2. Ujjayi Breath (Cobra Breathing)

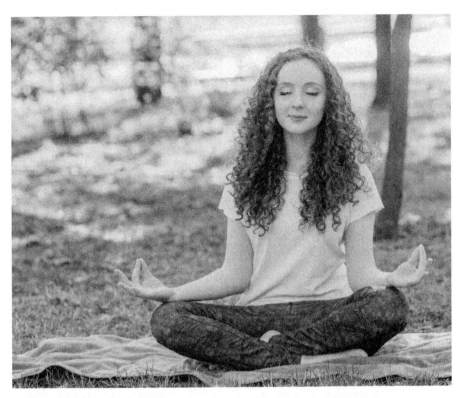

Ujjayi Breath is helpful to both energize and calm the body before a yoga session.

It is a pranayama that comprises inhaling through the nose, closing the mouth and keeping the inhalation, and then exhaling through the nose. Both inhalation and exhalation create a sound due to a mild contraction of the back of the throat, both deep and long and regulated. It's definitely the pranayama that is taught the most since it's very simple to perform and is effective.

Benefits:

· Raises the volume of oxygen in the blood.

· Builds internal heat in the body.

· Relieves tension.

• Promotes the free movement of prana.

• Regulates blood pressure.

• Allows sustaining a flow while practicing.

• Builds up energy.

• Detoxifies the body and mind.

• Promotes sensations of presence, self-awareness, and meditation.

How to Do:

1. Sit in Easy Pose (Cross-Legged).

2. **Mudra:** In Gyan Mudra, rest your palms on your knees with your thumb and index fingers touching, and other fingers extended. This generates a circuit that guides the prana to the brain.

3. Seal your lips and start breathing in and out of your nose.

4. Inhale through the nose, which is somewhat deeper than normal. Then, slowly exhale from your nose while constricting the muscles in the back of your throat.

5. If you have trouble getting the correct sound for your breath, try this:

   • Attempt to exhale the "HAAAH" sound with your mouth open—it's close to the tone you make when you're attempting to fog up a mirror. Get familiar with the sound so you can get the hang of the practice.

   • Close your mouth and try a similar sound, hearing the outflow of air through your nasal passages. Once you've mastered this on the outflow, use the same for in-flow breath, softly constricting the back of your throat as you inhale.

6. If you perform this properly, you will sound like waves in the ocean—the inhales can be related to the sound the ocean creates

when the water collects to form the wave, and the exhales can be compared to the sound of waves falling to the shore.

Drishti: Fix your gaze at the Third Eye Chakra (Between the brows).

Contradictions:

• When doing Ujjayi Pranayama, be cautious not to tighten your throat.

Timing: Keep doing that for as many breaths as you need to get to your core and settle. (At least 3 minutes.)

3. Sheetali Breath (Cooling Breath)

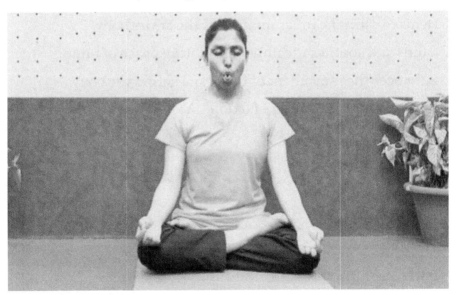

Sheetali Pranayama, also known as Cooling Breath, is a breathing activity that cools the body, mind, and emotions rapidly. Sheetali derives from the Sanskrit root "Sheet," which means frigid or cold. Sheetali translates literally as 'still, enthusiastic, and calming.'

In this pranayama, the inhalation is done through the tongue—like a tube—through doing Kunbhaka and then by exhaling the air through the nostrils. This pranayama was intended to lower body temperature. It can also be practiced when conducting Jalandhara and Mula Bandhas during retention.

Benefits:

· Balances excess Pitta.

· Cools the body and reduces unnecessary heat.

· Strengthens the digestive fire and encourages optimal digestion.

· Mitigates hyperacidity of the digestive tract.

· Relieves inflammatory skin disorders.

· Helps to calm the inflammation of the entire body.

· Calms and soothes the mind, promoting peace of mind.

· Enhances the movement of the prana across the body.

· Promotes a feeling of satisfaction.

· Fights fever.

· Relieves colicky pain.

· Enhances immunity.

· Relieves excess hunger.

· Triggers excess thirst.

· Decreases blood pressure.

How to Do:

1. Choose a cool, peaceful place where you will not be bothered. Prepare a steady, relaxed seat and balance the weight between the sitz bones, lengthen the back, and close the eyes. Rest your hands on your knees, palms facing up.

2. **Mudra:** In Gyan Mudra, put your hands on your knees. Close your eyes and curl up your tongue to form it like a tube.

3. Start with a body scan. Specifically, analyze which Pitta qualities are present in your body-mind (for example, excess heat, sharpness, oiliness, irritation, or intensity).

4. Practice Sheetali by inhaling through the curled tongue and exhaling through the nose. At each exhalation, gently tap the tip of the tongue on the roof of the mouth, welcoming the cold tip of the tongue to transfer coolness to the upper palate. Swallow now and then if your throat seems dry, repeat the cycle for 1-5 minutes—until you feel refreshed.

5. If you cannot curl your tongue, perform a variant known as Sitkari Pranayama (Inhale through your teeth, with your lips parted and your tongue floating right behind your teeth).

6. Pause and notice the effects of the activity, noting any parts of the body-mind that feel cleaned, ventilated, refreshed, or cooled.

7. Finish with a few minutes of silent meditation to indulge in the sensations of spaciousness.

Drishti: Focus your Drishti at the tip of your nose.

Contradictions:

• Since this practice requires inhalation from the mouth (which may not have the filtration potential of the nasal passages), it cannot be done if there is serious environmental pollution.

Timing: 3-5 minutes

4. Bhastrika Pranayama (Bellows Breath)

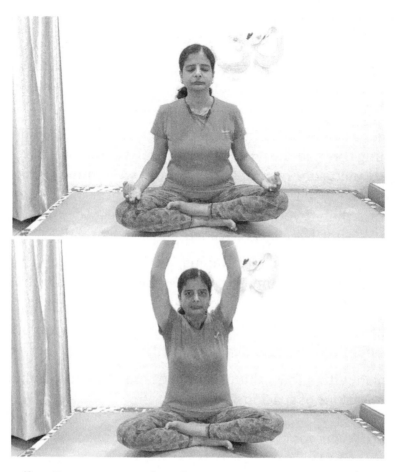

Bhastrika Pranayama, also known as Bellows Breath, is a warming breathing practice that mimics fanning a fire with a constant flow of air. "Bhastrika" is a Sanskrit term meaning "Bellows," which explains the successful filling and emptying of the abdomen and lungs during this practice. Bhastrika Pranayama activates the inner fire of mind and body, promoting proper digestion at all times.

Bhastrika is identical to Vatakrama Kapalabhati, but in Bhastrika both inhalation and exhalation are equal. It helps to fix any imbalances in the three doshas—Vata, Pitta, and Kapha. It is balancing for Kapha and Vata but should be practiced in moderation (and more gently) if Pitta is aggravated.

Benefits:

· It's fantastic for brain oxygenation.

· It benefits the nervous system and the motor system.

· It's perfect to energize the mind and body.

· Great for those suffering from depression and anxiety.

· Helps in treating fibrosis.

· Good for lungs and people suffering from repetitive cough, flu, respiratory infections, allergies, or breathlessness.

· Helps to improve immunity.

· Checks sleep apnea, too.

How to Do:

1. Sit in Vajrasana or Sukhasana (Cross-Legged Pose).

2. **Mudra:** Bring your hands to Gyan Mudra.

3. Inhale deeply, lifting your hands and opening your fists.

4. Exhale slightly, lowering your arms down next to your shoulders and closing your fists.

5. Keep going for 20 breaths.

6. Relax with your palms on your thighs.

7. Take a couple of normal breaths.

8. Keep going for two more rounds.

Drishti: Internal gaze; observe the sensations in your body in the present moment.

Contradictions:

· Make sure you do it on an empty stomach.

· Breastfeeding women should avoid this.

• Do this at your own pace. If you feel dizzy, extend the length of the break.

• If you suffer from hypertension and panic disorders, do it under the supervision of a teacher.

Timing: 3-5 minutes

5. Bhramari Breath (Humming Bee Breath)

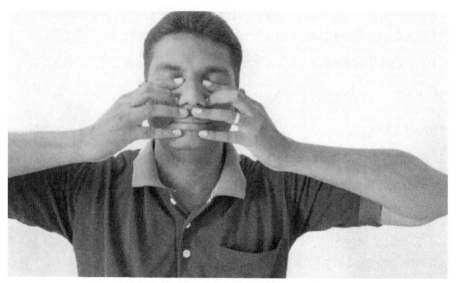

Bhramari Pranayama or Bumblebee Breath is a relaxing pranayama that can be practiced anywhere. Bhramari is derived from the Sanskrit word "Bee." This breathing method is named after the type of black Indian bee due to the bee-like buzzing sound created during the exhalation, others may say the sound of a hummingbird. This practice of breathing will relieve stress, agitation, and anger. It will even help to relax the mind and body before sleeping.

Benefits:

• Immediate release from tension, frustration, and anxiety. It is a very powerful breathing method for people suffering from hypertension since it soothes the anxious mind.

• Provides relief whether you feel hot or have a mild headache.

• Aims to reduce migraines.

• Helps in enhancing attention and memory.

• Builds confidence.

• Helps in the lowering of blood pressure.

• Aims to relax the mind to prepare for meditation.

How to Do:

1. Sit straight in a quiet, well-ventilated corner with your eyes closed. Keep a soft smile on your face.

2. Observe the sensations of the body and the quietness within.

3. **Mudra:** Shanmukhi Mudra (Close your eyes and cover your ears with your thumbs, your eyes with your index fingers, and your nose with your middle fingers. Press your upper lip slightly over your lower lip with your ring and little fingers).

4. Take a deep breath and press the cartilage softly as you breathe out. You should keep the cartilage squeezed or press it in and out with the fingers while making a loud humming sound like a bee.

5. You may produce a low-pitched sound, too, but it's a smart choice to make a high-pitched sound for better results.

6. Breathe in again and follow the same pattern 3-4 times.

Drishti: Focus on the Third Eye Chakra, between the eyebrows.

Contradiction:

• None. Anybody from an infant to an aged individual can perform this pranayama. The only condition is that this pranayama should be performed on an empty stomach.

Timing: 3-5 minutes

Meditation

Trataka Sadhana (Fixed Gazing Meditation)

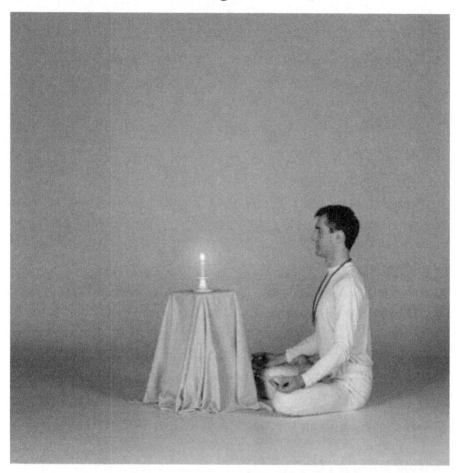

In Hatha Yoga, apart from asanas and pranayamas, 'Shatkarmas' are also included. Trataka is one of the Shat Kriyas (Six Yogic Cleansing Processes).

Trataka is a yogic purification and a tantric form of meditation that includes looking at a specific point, such as a tiny point, a black dot, or a candle flame. It is believed to bring energy to the "Third Eye" (Ajna Chakra) and to promote different spiritual abilities.

Through fixing the gaze, the distracted mind comes to a halt. It is often claimed that the control of the ciliary (blink) reflex activates the pineal gland, which Kundalini Yoga associates with the Third Eye. Trataka is said to improve the capacity to concentrate. It increases the power of memory and puts the mind into a state of awareness, attention, and focus.

Benefits:

• Improves our concentration.

• Calms our restless mind.

• Promotes emotional stability.

• It may raise your overall frequency.

• Boosts our willpower.

• Develops insight and clairvoyance.

• Improves our consciousness power.

• Trataka helps in activating the Kundalini.

• It helps you with balanced left and right brain functions.

• Purifies the eyes, strengthens the muscles of the eyes, and improves vision and memory.

• Helps with sleeping issues and bed-wetting.

• Strengthens the ability to focus, which is advised for school children.

• Develops intuition, the capacity to visualize, and willpower.

• Practice balances the nervous system and relieves stress, anxiety, depression, and insomnia.

• Since the blinking of the eye is under our control as we focus our attention on the tiny objects of any material, it helps us improve our eye muscles.

• As we stare at an object such as a candle flame or some other tiny object, it increases the concentration power of our eyes and cures eye disorders.

• Practicing Trataka brings us peace by extracting harmful feelings and urges from our heads. This allows us to relieve insomnia.

• It will increase your awareness and connect you to live at a higher spiritual and soul level.

• It improves your emotional intelligence and psychic abilities.

• Trataka Meditation can activate your Third Eye.

How to Do:

1. Light the candle and position it at the level of the eye, ensuring that it does not flicker.

2. Sit in a relaxed meditative pose with your hands on your knees in Gyan or Chin Mudra. Set an intention or simply breathe to calm your body and develop stillness.

3. Close your eyes and open them, aiming at the center of the candle flame, right above the wick. Try to hold your eyes steady without blinking.

4. Gaze as long as you can without straining your eyes and then shut them when you need to.

5. Look to the center of the eyebrows with your eyes closed. Continue to hold the picture of the flame in your awareness for as long as possible, concentrate on it and observe any colors that may appear.

6. When the picture fades, repeat the procedure and continue for 5-10 minutes.

7. If the mind wanders, focus on the breath, imagining the breath rushing in and out of the Third Eye.

Drishti: Point your gaze at the center of the flame.

Contradictions:

• This activity is not appropriate for those with psychic disorders.

• Those who have a propensity to schizophrenia or hallucinations should not practice Trataka.

Timing: 5-10 minutes

Ends the session by putting your hands together in Prayer Pose over your heart, bowing and thanking god for this life and everything.

I know the session feels never-ending, thus you can always let go of some asanas and perform the ones you like; a few well-performed asanas are any day better than 10s of poorly performed asanas. Just don't break the sequence.

BEST PRACTICES TO AVOID INJURY

While yoga has several benefits, yoga injuries can occur when individuals push themselves too hard and too fast. Some of the most common yoga injuries include pulls or strains in the neck, spine, lower back, or hamstring.

Yoga postures more likely to cause injuries are a Headstand or Handstand (inversions), backbends like Locust or Wheel Pose, Shoulder Stand, and often bending too much or too far to one side.

If you are in good health, Hatha Yoga is usually healthy, although as with any other form of exercise, there are certain safety measures to keep in mind.

Following these 10 simple rules listed below will help ensure that you avoid injury and have a satisfying, healthy, and safe Hatha Yoga session.

1. Practice Yoga Cautiously (Especially If You're a Beginner)

Don't assume that you should be able to bend or move in ways other students can. Everyone is different, so "Perfect Postural Alignment" may not be possible for you in some yoga poses. Even if an instructor really pressures you, forces you down, or puts pressure to get you further into a pose than you are comfortable with, make sure you ask them to back off.

2. Set a Goal Before Each Practice

A goal such as having realistic expectations or not competing (with yourself or others) leads you through the practice with ease. Setting a goal establishes the basis for each practice that you may return to throughout. If you start to feel distracted or off course, you can check in and re-center your goal.

3. Use Props for Support

Props, including yoga blocks, straps, blankets, and even a wall or chair can really come in handy. These are especially helpful for a newbie in yoga, the elderly, or those healing from injuries.

Using a rolled blanket under your hips will help you with postures like Pigeon Pose or other hip flexor openers. If the hands don't reach the floor in a forward bend, side bend, or twist, use blocks on the floor to 'bring the mat closer' and take pressure on the legs as you bend over. Straps are helpful when you lie on your back and stretch your legs; just don't pull too hard or too fast. Also, feel free to consult a teacher for advice on the use of props if you have limitations.

4. Yoga is about Listening to Your Body

To reduce the possibility of injuries while doing yoga, stop forcing yourself too hard into postures that hurt or are contraindicated based on your abilities.

Recognizing pain and honoring your body enough to back off will prevent injury. There is a line between power and force. Use your breath and presence to be powerful in your pose without forcing your body beyond its capabilities.

5. Stretch Tight Areas Gently

Stretching should always be performed thoughtfully, gently, and slowly. Take your time loosening tight areas—such as hips, calves, or hamstrings—to be careful not to move too quickly into any poses.

Remember to warm up the body before any intense exercise with some stretching, as this tends to relax muscles that might be susceptible to tension. It's safe to experience mild to moderate discomfort when stretching or bending, just be cautious not to exceed the boundaries. Overstretching is always damaging, as it can worsen existing injuries and lead to tears, pulls, and other pains.

6. Do Not Compete with Yourself

Develop the attitude of non-competition with yourself. First and foremost, listen to your body. While it's enjoyable to attempt challenging poses, it's not worth the risk of injury if you don't feel up to it on a given occasion.

7. Get Your Doctor's Advice if You Have Any Injuries

Even though Hatha Yoga is safe and fun for just about anyone, I recommend that you should always consult your doctor before beginning a new regimen. If you have elevated blood pressure, are susceptible to seizures, are pregnant or have some other medical problems, had intolerance problems in the past, then it is best to make sure that the doctor is on board before you start practicing.

Also, work with a physical therapist or a personal trainer for support at first if you have any existing injuries before beginning a yoga practice. Ask for references or instructor advice, get clearance to start a new style if it appears to be vigorous (such as Ashtanga or Bikram), and ask if there are yoga types you should avoid. You should also get guidance from the orthopedic or chiropractor if you are still uncertain of which postures and movements can be dangerous due to your limitations.

8. Don't Compete

There is no competition in yoga. This is your opportunity to practice a relaxed body, breath, and mental awareness. Be gentle, yet firm with your body. Do not pressure or surpass your ability.

9. Do Not Aggravate Any Current Health Problems

Use common sense. Refrain from any practice that might cause pain, suffering, or mental anxiety. Common medical symptoms or conditions requiring caution include high blood pressure, stomach ulcer, hernia, lower back pain, spinal disc problems, pregnancy, etc.

10. Cautions for Women

It is not recommended that you practice inverted yoga postures during your menstrual period.

These points are not to scare you, but to make you more aware so that you don't end up hurting yourself. Yoga should be fun and challenging. Following these tips will launch you off the mat and into your life with strength and energy, not pain.

Just remember to stay hydrated and listen to your body; don't push yourself, and take a break (or walk out) if you feel lightheaded or unwell.

BEGINNERS COMMON MISTAKES AND HOW TO FIX THEM

No one begins being great at yoga, it requires time and practice. And part of this process involves learning from mistakes. Here are some of the most common Hatha Yoga mistakes:

1. Not Doing Warm-Up

Warm-up postures such as light twisting and bending, shoulder rotation, and spinal rocking, help you prepare for the upcoming activities. You're enhancing muscle flexibility, loosening regions of the body, increasing blood supply to the extremities, and concentrating your attention on the task ahead. All-in-all, a warm-up routine is just as critical as the yoga practice itself.

The other reason to do a warm-up before you start your yoga session is that before you practice, warming up allows you to rediscover your body's consciousness and interact with your breath. Therefore, always warm up before you start your Hatha Yoga session (1-2 rounds of Sun Salutation is enough).

2. Not Dressing Appropriately

Clothes that are too tight, restricting, scratchy, or sweaty will distract you from focusing on your practice. Thus, wear loose clothes that can be easily carried and made of fabrics that feel good on your skin.

Consider what makes you comfortable performing your Sun Salutations (Surya Namaskar) and base your clothing decisions on that. Shorts, cropped pants, leggings, or slightly flared yoga pants are just fine. For men, lightweight joggers and cotton or polyester t-shirts will do fine.

If you need any guidance on what to wear, you can always ask the front desk staff of the particular yoga studio for guidance.

3. Letting Your Eyes Wander around the Room

"Drishti or focused gaze," is when your eyes are aimed at a certain point in your yoga practice. Setting a physical point to focus on is an important component of finding presence, balance, and mid-flow power; this tactic also helps to focus . It's easy to get distracted by thoughts or someone's presence, but focusing at a point during each pose will bring your focus to the mind, breath, and practice.

4. Not Hydrating Enough

Dehydration is a significant source of stress and emotional imbalances. Children are 90% water and adults are 70 % water. Drinking enough fluids—water (not juice, pop, or coffee)—is essential to allow your body to naturally keep in balance and heal itself.

5. Not Letting Your Breath Flow Freely

Most of us don't know how to breathe. We take short breaths as if we were afraid of breathing. We should practice breathing deeply to rejuvenate and feed our bodies.

Breath is the ideal resource to attain physical and mental peace and to find a proper expression of the pose. Iyengar Yoga uses various pranayamas to affect breathing and control various states of consciousness, relaxation, and well-being.

6. Not Utilizing the Proper Environment

Hatha Yoga can be done anywhere. But it's best to find a quiet, distraction-free space that has a comfortable (not too hot, not too cool) environment. This should be a spot that you find peaceful and where you are not likely to be bothered. It could be a place where you gather your favorite things. Keep a bottle of water beside you.

7. Practicing with a Full Stomach

It's best to perform yoga on an empty stomach, so don't eat at least 2-3 hours before the practice. Since Hatha Yoga uses several breathing exercises (pranayamas), movements (asanas), and meditation, it can be uncomfortable with a full stomach.

But feeling like you're starving isn't nice either. Escape disturbances from fullness and hunger by having a light snack an hour or two before your Hatha Yoga session begins. I recommend following a diet that includes complete, basic, and fresh food, without having meat and eggs.

8. Getting Mixed Up between Cobra Pose and Upward-Facing Dog

Students tend to do neither Cobra Pose nor Upward-Facing Dog, and instead do some in-between pose. The most crucial difference between Cobra Pose and Upward-Facing Dog is that in Cobra Pose you utilize the strength of your spine to get up while in Upward-Facing Dog you use your hands.

Your legs and pelvis are well off the floor in Upward-Facing Dog while in Cobra Pose, your legs, pelvis, and even your lower ribs stay on the floor with your elbows bent to help lengthen your spine.

9. Making the Practice Complicated

Hatha Yoga is all about long-holding asanas, pranayamas,

relaxation, and meditation. The aim is to develop physical vitality and raise awareness. But with the overwhelming amount of asanas, it's easy to get carried away.

I insist you start with a few simple, comfortable ones of your choice; later you can add more asanas to your sequence. You're also allowed to use props if you need.

Always remember, less is more. Two well-performed asanas with enough time to settle in are more beneficial than half a dozen fast or poorly-performed ones.

10. Keeping your Phone with You

Why should you have something in your soothing space that has been shown to trigger depression and anxiety? Allow yourself an hour without your phone. It disturbs your peace of mind.

11. Not Setting an End Goal to the Practice

'Sankalpa' is the Sanskrit word for intention. Setting your intention to practice yoga is simply bringing your focus to the quality that you would like to achieve with your time on and off the mat. This quality may be gratitude, strength, awareness—whatever you choose to cultivate.

Although people who begin doing any form of yoga are more likely to do so for a specific purpose, many don't set a specific intention for the practice; it's like they're on the bike with no direction. So, determine what you're hoping to accomplish and set your own realistic goals.

12. Not Following the Sequence

Sure, you can deduct some asanas but do not alter the order. Hatha Yoga is a science to bring about a specific outcome. Don't mess with what works. Always start with the warm-up and end with a calming meditation session, following the sequence.

13. Going into a Deep Pose Too Fast

This advice is not solely for beginners. Once you step into a forward fold, you may want to touch your toes rapidly. Yet what is much more effective and safer is to continue with a relaxed variant of the pose, with your hands on your thighs. Then after a couple of breaths, gradually move towards the toes. That way, you can make greater improvements with your flexibility, and you will avoid the risk of harming yourself as well.

14. Not Modifying the Practice

When you rest more, you can have the temptation to alter the poses to make you feel more stable and rooted. This can be achieved in a variety of poses by lowering a knee in the lunge, for example, by using supports on the inside of the leg instead of the outside. Resting and modifying in the practice is a sign of a mature student; one who listens to his/her inner self.

15. Not Taking Proper Post-Yoga Meals

With adequate hydration before and after practice, the nutrition you take after the session would be a welcoming experience over a ravenous attack on food and drink. Keep away from alcohol and stick with a healthy balance of protein, carbohydrates, and foods that are easy to digest. Foods like brown rice and vegetables, rice sushi, or grilled vegetables are some perfect choices.

16. Not Stopping Right Away

If you start to feel light-headed, dizzy, or nauseous, there's no shame in taking a break and getting some water.

It's important to bear in mind that the practice of yoga is meant to improve the awareness of the body at this present moment. If your body cries out for water or rest, listen to it. You're your best friend in the yoga session and in general. Hatha Yoga may be extremely helpful to practice, but as with any form of physical activity, you need to be careful and safe.

17. Forgetting to Stabilize Your Core

By pulling the pit of your belly in and up towards your spine, you will naturally neutralize the pelvis and the lower back to make every pose stronger and safer. When you let your core fall which may cause you to arch your lower back, it puts pressure on your lower back. So, always brace your core by bringing your belly button to your spine and stabilizing your abs.

18. Thinking that Props are for Inexperienced

Blocks, straps, blankets, balls, towels, chairs, walls, sandbags, eye bags, and pillows are all considered fair play to assist you in yoga because the body comes first. When you ignore props, the muscles need to make up for the extra effort. The more you pressurize your muscle, the less you will relax.

The more thoroughly the body is supported, the stronger the feeling of peace and surrender would be. So, support your body as much as you can—your body will reward you with deep sighs of relaxation. Plus, props will help us enter the pose and hit the correct area of the body. They will help us move deeper into a pose and protect us from injuries.

19. Not Doing the Pose on the Other Side

Make sure to perform the pose on both sides. Hold the pose on both sides for the same period of time.

20. Taking It Too Easy

While Hatha Yoga appears easy, it can be difficult for beginners. Just because the body rests comfortably doesn't mean the mind will relax into stillness, too. Be patient, and be prepared for the days when you just don't want to do it anymore.

With time and practice, you will be rewarded with the ability to move effortlessly to a place of deep contentment. After all, that is what yoga is all about—holding our fidgety bodies still and soothing our turbulent minds so that we can relax peacefully in the present moment and see the hidden peace that resides within.

21. Not Being Regular

Do not expect overnight results or feel that you must master any practice quickly. Results will come in a surprisingly short time of their own accord, but you'll have to be regular in your practice.

22. Not Enjoying It!

OK, the last beginner's mistake is, not enjoying it. Really, have fun! Take it all in, don't fret, and enjoy the experience. I want you to love it!

COMMON MYTHS AND FAQS

13 Common Myths

Myth #1: Hatha Yoga is Easy

Hatha may be a great introduction to yoga, but should not be mistaken for "Easy" yoga. It can still be challenging both physically and mentally. Hatha Yoga sessions provide a venue for stretching, relaxing, and easing stress—essential to both busy lives and recovery following intense workouts.

Myth #2: Spiritual Body is a Myth

The spiritual body is real! It can take any form. There is no death or degradation in this divine entity. The body of the soul is immortal. This spiritual body is like the subatomic particles, neither formed nor demolished, except to change their outward appearance.

Myth #3: It Doesn't Help with Anxiety

Meditation is a technique that cleanses the mind and extracts junk from the mind. The Hatha Yoga meditation will allow you to remove conscious and subconscious fears that trigger tension, worry, and anxiety. Yoga's many emotional gains are remarkable—from less anxiety and greater focus to higher self-esteem and more fulfilling intimate relationships.

Myth #4: I Have to be a Certain Way to Do Yoga

There are no requirements for practicing yoga. You don't need to be stronger, skinnier, more flexible, or physically fit than you are now. There are many styles to choose from depending on what you're heading to yoga for. Yoga has something for everyone, and the good news is that there is no downside to yoga. If you listen to your body and go at your own pace, you'll soon see what yoga has to offer you.

Myth #5: Yoga is Just for Women

Yoga is for everyone. While it may be true that most classes are filled by women majority, more and more men are finding the practice. In fact, many of the traditional founders of yoga in India were men!

Whether you are male or female, yoga offers a physical challenge, a mental challenge, and the opportunity to experience a wide range of health benefits. From physical therapists to medical doctors—regarding disease prevention techniques, injury rehabilitation, stress reduction, and overall health—yoga is highly recommended.

Myth #6: Hatha Yoga Don't Help You Lose Weight

While Hatha Yoga may not be as successful as a cardio session or more rigorous yoga practice like Ashtanga or Bikram in weight loss, a combination of 1-hour of Hatha Yoga a day with the avoidance of a few hundred calories from your diet will contribute to a gradual, steady, and healthy weight loss.

Myth #7: Yoga is Out of My Budget

Most studios offer monthly specials for unlimited Yoga classes and Pilates classes, lowering the average cost to about $8 per class. Yoga isn't a splurge—it's an expenditure on your health, well-being, and peace of mind.

And if you choose to practice Hatha Yoga at home, it'd be even cheaper; you'll just need a yoga mat, blankets and blocks for support (optional), and a water bottle.

Myth #8: I'm TOO Sick to Do Yoga

Yoga sessions heal you from the inside out when you practice it regularly. Yogis get sick less and hardly ever have chronic illnesses. The average yogi spends about 1% of his/her income on health issues, compared to 26% or more for non-yogis.

Myth #9: Yoga and Music Go Well

When you practice asanas, there should never be any music. Hatha Yoga demands the involvement of your body, mind, energy, and the innermost core. If you want to get connected in what is the source of existence within you, your body, mind, and energy need to be thoroughly involved. You should approach it with a certain respect and focus. Not just going through it playing music.

One of the major challenges in yoga studios is that the instructor is performing asanas and communicating. This is a sure means of harming oneself. The breath, mental focus, and stability of energy are most important when you are doing the asana. If you speak, you will destroy all that.

Myth #10: I'm TOO Old to Do Yoga

You're never too old to perform yoga as gentle as Hatha. The older you get, the better you can do them. It does not demand much movement and can be immensely helpful to old people.

Myth #11: Yoga Takes Plenty of Time

You may need to set aside 40-120 minutes for a Hatha Yoga session, so on one hand this is true, but on the other hand, you will gain precious "Me-Time" as you experience feelings of happiness and overall well-being. The physical, mental, and spiritual effects of it will motivate you to become a stronger person. So, yoga doesn't take time, it gives you your "Me-Time."

Myth #12: Yoga Should be Practiced Every Morning and Evening

Yoga isn't something you need to do morning-evening. It's a way of being. One has to become 'Yoga.'

No aspect of life is excluded from the yogic process. If your life becomes 'Yoga,' then you can do everything. You can run your family, you can go to the office, you can run your business, and you can do whatever you want with no issues if your way of being becomes 'Yoga.' Every aspect of life, either you can use to entangle yourself or to free yourself. If you use it to entangle yourself, we call it 'Karma.' If you're using it to liberate yourself, we call it 'Yoga.'

Myth #13: Yoga Comes from Hinduism and is a Religion

The word "Hindu" has come from the word "Sindhu", which is a river. Because this culture grew from the banks of the river Sindhu or Indus, this culture got labeled as Hindu. Hindu is not an "ism"—it is not a religion. It is a geographical and cultural identity.

Yoga has nothing to do with religion and is based on the science of mind-body connection. Saying 'Yoga' is Hindu is like saying 'Gravity' is Christian. Just because the law of gravity was propounded by Isaac Newton, who lived in a Christian culture, does it make gravity Christian? Yoga is a technology. All people of all religious backgrounds are welcome to practice yoga and enjoy the benefits yoga can offer to the mind, body, and soul.

20 Common FAQs

1. Why Should I Do Hatha Yoga?

Hatha Yoga is a thousand-year-old yogic practice that people are still adapting to achieve overall body and mind health. People focus on the physical body, including stressing the chakras to stimulate Kundalini and facilitate spiritual and physical well-being, including the elimination of diseases.

With the practice of Hatha Yoga, an individual can balance his mind, body, and chakras and learn controlled meditation and breathing techniques. These techniques complement the body's physical movements. The basic aspect of Hatha Yoga is the "Hatha Yoga Pradipika," the yogic practice that is rooted in Hindu yoga. The text of Hatha Yoga is the "Svatmarama Hatha Yoga Pradipika," which is the official text of Hatha Yoga. It says that Hatha Yoga is a way to ascend to the highest form of Raja Yoga that will make you shine effortlessly.

2. I Can't Do the Postures Perfectly; Will I Still Get the Benefits?

It's not important how far you can get into the yoga pose. What's crucial is that you do the pose with the proper orientation of your body—put all your energy into the pose while still breathing and holding your head relaxed. There is no comparable standard in yoga.

3. What is the Difference between Hatha Yoga and Other Yoga Styles?

Hatha Yoga focuses on perfecting asanas and doing pranayama to increase the flow of vital energy throughout the body. Hatha works, in particular, to improve the flow of energy through meditation. While Ashtanga and other active yoga styles still contain these components, the poses flow more dynamically.

4. Can I Practice Hatha Yoga When Pregnant?

Prenatal Yoga, Hatha Yoga, and Restorative Yoga are the best choices for pregnant women. Usually, it's okay to proceed as usual during the first trimester, but you can always consult a midwife or a doctor just to make sure.

5. How can Hatha Yoga Relieve Stress?

Yoga encourages us to take some time for ourselves. It's a well-known fact that exercise and meditation relieve stress, and the Hatha Yoga curriculum delivers the same commitment and more.

The stretching and strengthening of yoga recharge and strengthen the body, and the inner awareness of yogic breathing and meditation calms the mind. When the body is relaxed and healthy and the mind is centered and calm, we are motivated to meet the complexities of life with freshness and courage.

So, the natural way to avoid stress is to turn up on a yoga mat and do some Hatha Yoga poses. Every Hatha Yoga asana guides us to peace of mind and positivity.

6. How Often Should I Practice Hatha Yoga?

To get started, it is helpful to commit to practice 1-3 times a week for some weeks and then re-evaluate. This puts you in the habit and lets you get physical gains and positive improvements in your awareness. Practicing once a week can even have a positive impact on your everyday life.

7. What Should I Bring to the Yoga Session?

Wear loose, comfortable clothes. Carry a mat, water bottle, a soft pillow or some blocks for support (optional), and a light blanket for meditation and relaxation at the end of the session (optional). The most important thing is to carry your Joyful Spirit!

8. Who Should Avoid Doing Hatha Yoga?

Hatha Yoga is safe and appropriate for individuals of all age groups. However, there are a few precautions that need to be taken before you participate in this practice, especially if you have any chronic illnesses. This practice should be avoided by people with a history of glaucoma, cardiovascular disease, and sciatica.

9. What Do I Wear?

Wear loose clothes that can be easily carried and made of fabrics that feel good on your skin. Consider what makes you comfortable performing your Sun Salutations (Surya Namaskar) and base your clothing decisions on that. Shorts, cropped pants, leggings, or slightly flared yoga pants are just fine. For men, lightweight joggers and cotton or polyester t-shirts will do fine.

If you need any guidance on what to wear, you can always ask the front desk staff of the particular yoga studio for guidance.

10. How am I Supposed to Prepare for a Hatha Yoga Session?

Perform Hatha Yoga on an empty stomach; if not, eat two hours before your session starts and be well-hydrated.

11. Can Hatha Yoga Help Lower Back Problems?

The heat produced by different asanas in the session warms the body and allows the joints to move more smoothly. The sequence of breathing techniques and poses is designed to create strength across the entire body, particularly through the back. If practiced regularly, you'll quickly notice an increased range of motion and pain reduction in your daily life.

12. Am I TOO Old for Hatha Yoga?

Yin Yoga and Hatha Yoga are great yoga styles that can be incorporated into your yoga curriculum as you grow older. This is because these types of yoga focus especially on joint health and breathing.

13. How Much Water Should I Drink Before the Session?

"Be well-hydrated!" Before the session, I suggest that you drink about 2-3 liters of water (not just prior to the session but slowly starting as you wake up to the time you start the session).

14. Can I Drink Water during the Session?

You can drink any time during your session, of course. Your body needs about 30 minutes to process water into your bloodstream, so it's better to stay properly hydrated and not dependent on hydration class sips. Also, filling yourself with liquid, then moving your body back, forward, upside down, and so on can make you feel a little sick. Always keep a water bottle with you. If you need to refill on a rare occasion, please seek to do so between asanas, not during.

15. Should I Eat Before the Session?

It's best to perform Hatha Yoga on an empty stomach, so don't eat at least 2-3 hours before practice. Since Hatha Yoga uses several pranayamas, asanas, and meditation, it can be painful and distracting with a full stomach. A small snack (a piece of fruit or a handful of nuts) is fine an hour or so before.

16. Can I Do Yoga If I Eat Non-Veg and Drink?

As per Sadhguru, *'Yoga isn't a restriction, it's a deeper understanding of life. If you knew how to become absolutely ecstatic just by your own chemistry, you wouldn't smoke or take a drink in your life. I've never touched a substance but if you look at my eyes, I'm always stoned. Yogis look at alcohol, drugs, and these things as kindergarten stuff because we can get intoxicated a thousand times over just with our aliveness. Why simply wine? You can get drunk with the di-vine!'*

17. When Will I Start to See Results?

How quickly you progress will depend entirely on you—to a small extent on your natural ability, but mostly on the honest time and effort you put into your yoga practice. It's going to require regular hard work and practice. You will reap the physical, mental, and spiritual benefits of this activity gradually, but don't expect to see results right away.

18. How Long Do I Need to Practice for Each Day?

Any amount of time you spent on your practice would offer major benefits. You might start with just ½ an hour in the evenings, and once you notice the obvious benefits, you'll be inspired to practice longer. But don't rush the practice, whatever you do; various asanas are quick enough to fit into your time. Even a 3-minute meditation pays off when you practice regularly.

Take your time, enjoy each pose, and allow yourself the luxury of a relaxation period, even if it's only a few minutes. Relaxing in and loving the practice to the utmost is key to having all the advantages that can accumulate over time.

19. Do I Need to Abstain from Sex to Rise My Kundalini?

You can get the idea of how powerful your semen or ovum can be by the fact that it can give rise to a new being; that's the power of it! As per ancient Indian Rishis, a drop of semen comprises 40 *drops* of bone marrow, and 40 drops of blood make a drop of bone marrow. I highly urge you to save your vital fluid if you're on the path of self-discovery and spiritual growth. It has done wonders for me and will definitely change your life. The energy, confidence, and benefits are beyond words, especially for anyone seeking spiritual goals.

Celibacy will offer a fresh light and perspective into the spiritual path. The joy of getting married or merged with God or Goddess isn't just a vow. Instead, the road is sparkling with optimism and love. He/she who wishes to lift his or her consciousness level from the lower chakras to the top of the head really has no choice.

By practicing celibacy, you provide each chakra the newness

of Kundalini's upward stroke. The Kundalini rises as if a great artist was painting an upward stroke on a blank canvas. Nothing flows downward. It's all flowing up. The help you get when you follow celibacy is beyond the understanding of the human imagination.

20. When to Practice?

Yoga is ideally practiced at the same time every day, to encourage the discipline of the practice. It can be done at any time of the day. Some prefer it as a wake-up routine in the morning, while others like to wind down and de-stress with yoga at the end of the day.

A REQUEST

Dear Reader,

As you near the conclusion of this book, I'd like to convey my heartfelt appreciation for sticking with me on this journey. I hope the pages you've read have inspired you, taught you insight, and sparked an interest in Hatha Yoga.

Please consider posting a review on Amazon to share your opinions and experiences. By sharing your review, you not only contribute to common knowledge but also have a significant ripple effect of change and healing in the lives of many readers. If this is an ebook, here is a link that'll take you directly to the review section- Click Here

Thank you for your presence, for your support, and for your willingness to start on this transforming journey. May the knowledge contained within these pages continue to resonate deep in your heart and lead you on your road to overall well-being.

Once again thanks for reading...

You can lend this book to your family, it's free of cost!!

You can also contact me for any queries: rohit@rohitsahu.net or on any of the following social media:

Facebook, Twitter, Instagram, Goodreads, Linkedin

Want to Hear from Me on Ayurveda and Spirituality? - https://rohitsahu.net/join-to-hear/

HERE ARE YOUR
FREE GIFTS!!

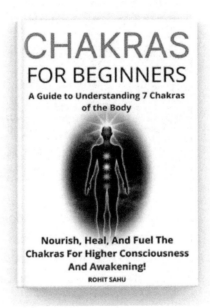

A basic introduction to the 7 Chakras... If you're into Chakras and pursuing knowledge about Chakras Awakening and Vibrational Energy, this book will help you pave the way towards your spiritual growth.

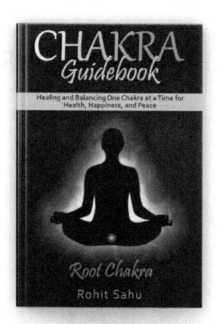

Your 1st Book in the "Chakra Guidebook" series is FREE! This is packed with all the information, tips, and techniques that will make sure that you can effectively heal, balance, and open your Root Chakra.

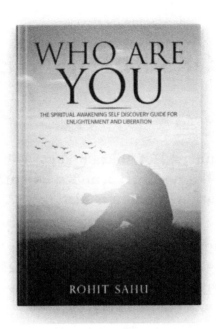

Have you ever thought after reaching your goal, why aren't you happy? It's because that is not what you need to be happy. This is not just another self-help book; this spiritual workbook will help you achieve liberation and be self-enlightened!

CLICK HERE to Claim the Books!!

BOOKS IN THIS SERIES

» Yoga For Beginners: Hot/Bikram Yoga: The Complete Guide To Master Hot/Bikram Yoga; Benefits, Essentials, Poses (With Pictures), Precautions, Common Mistakes, FAQs And Common Myths

» Yoga For Beginners: Iyengar Yoga: The Complete Guide to Master Iyengar Yoga; Benefits, Essentials, Asanas (with Pictures), Pranayamas, Meditation, Safety Tips, Common Mistakes, FAQs, and Common Myths

» Yoga For Beginners: Restorative Yoga: The Complete Guide To Master Restorative Yoga; Benefits, Essentials, Poses (With Pictures), Precautions, Common Mistakes, FAQs And Common Myths

» Yoga For Beginners: Power Yoga: The Complete Guide to Master Power Yoga; Benefits, Essentials, Poses (with Pictures), Precautions, Common Mistakes, FAQs, and Common Myths

» Yoga For Beginners: Vinyasa Yoga: The Complete Guide to Master Vinyasa Yoga; Benefits, Essentials, Asanas (with Pictures), Pranayamas, Safety Tips, Common Mistakes, FAQs, and Common Myths

» Yoga For Beginners: Kundalini Yoga: The Complete Guide to Master Kundalini Yoga; Benefits, Essentials, Kriyas (with Pictures), Kundalini Meditation, Common Mistakes, FAQs, and Common Myths

» Yoga For Beginners: Hatha Yoga: The Complete Guide to Master Hatha Yoga; Benefits, Essentials, Asanas (with Pictures), Hatha Meditation, Common Mistakes, FAQs, and

Common Myths

» Yoga For Beginners: Ashtanga Yoga: The Complete Guide to Master Ashtanga Yoga; Benefits, Essentials, Asanas (with Pictures), Ashtanga Meditation, Common Mistakes, FAQs, and Common Myths

» Yoga For Beginners: Prenatal Yoga: The Complete Guide to Master Prenatal Yoga; Benefits, Essentials, Pranayamas, Asanas (with Pictures), Common Mistakes, FAQs, and Common Myths

» Yoga For Beginners: Kripalu Yoga: The Complete Guide to Master Kripalu Yoga; Benefits, Essentials, Asanas (with Pictures), Pranayamas, Meditation, Safety Tips, Common Mistakes, FAQs, and Common Myths

BOOKS BY THIS AUTHOR

Ayurveda For Beginners (3 Book Series)

Ayurveda, which derives from ancient Vedic scriptures, is a 5,000-year-old medical ideology and philosophy based on the idea that we are all made up of different types of energy.

There are three Doshas in Ayurveda that describe the dominant state of mind/body: Vata, Pitta, and Kapha. While all three are present in everyone, Ayurveda suggests that we each have a dominant Dosha that is unwavering from birth, and ideally an equal (though often fluctuating) balance between the other two.

If Doshas are balanced, we are healthy; when they are unbalanced, we develop a disorder commonly expressed by skin problems, impaired nutrition, insomnia, irritability, and anxiety.

Vata, Pitta, and Kapha are all important to our biology in some way, so no one is greater than, or superior to, any other. Each has a very specific set of basic functions to perform in the body.

That said, when the Doshas are out of control, our wellbeing can be damaged. However, before we get into the particulars of each of the three Doshas, it is helpful to understand their basic nature and their wider function in the natural world.

Each of the Doshas has its own special strengths and weaknesses, and with a little awareness, you can do a lot to remain healthy and balanced. You can use this series to adjust your lifestyles and routines in a way that supports your constitution.

I've made a complete series of these three.

Just follow the books along, you'll reveal the easiest step-by-step routine to balance your Dosha by the end of it!

Ayurveda Cookbook For Beginners (3 Book Series)

All you need to know about Ayurvedic diet and cooking along with easy-to-follow recipes backed by the timeless wisdom of Indian heritage to balance your aggravated dosha...

I've made a complete cookbook series on all 3 doshas! You can use this series to adjust your lifestyles and routines in a way that supports your constitution.

With this "Ayurveda Cookbook For Beginners Series," I provide you the best dietary practices, recipes, and everything you need to balance and heal your doshas alongside enjoying the authentic Indian flavors.

This guide's Ayurvedic Cooking techniques tell what to eat and how to eat to help the healing process and assist the body in removing contaminants and maintaining equilibrium. It has a wealth of knowledge on healthy diet, proper food combinations, food quality, food timing, and cooking methods.

All the recipes in this cookbook are traditional, time-tested over decades, and are based on Ayurvedic principles. They can aid a yogi's yoga practice by keeping the mind calm and are thus ideal for all yoga practitioners. The beauty is that the recipes are not only sattvic in nature but are also tasty and have that authentic Indian taste!

Yoga For Beginners (10 Book Series)

Yoga origin can be traced back to more than 5,000 years ago, but some researchers believe that yoga may be up to 10,000 years old. The word 'Yoga' first appeared in the oldest sacred texts, the Rig Veda, and is derived from the Sanskrit root "Yuj" which means to unite.

According to the Yoga Scriptures, the practice of yoga leads an individual to a union of consciousness with that of universal consciousness. It eventually leads to a great harmony between the human mind and body, man, and nature.

Yoga provides multiple health advantages, such as enhancing endurance, reducing depression, and improving overall wellness and fitness.

As yoga has grown into mainstream popularity, many styles and variations have emerged in wellness space. This centuries-old Eastern philosophy is now widely practiced and taught by people of all ages, sizes, and backgrounds.

There are 10 primary types of Yoga. So if you're trying to figure out which of the different types of Yoga is best for you, remember that there's no one right or wrong. You can ask yourself what's important to you in your Yoga practice: Are you searching for a sweaty, intense practice, or are you searching for a more meditative, gentler practice that looks more appealing?

Like you choose any sort of exercise, choose something you want to do.

Here's a complete series on all 10 types of yoga.

This guide can be used by beginners, advanced students, teachers, trainees, and teacher training programs. Covering the fundamentals of each pose in exact detail, including how to correct the most common mistakes, as well as changes to almost all body types, this yoga guides has left nothing to help you make daily breakthroughs.

Ayurvedic Weight Loss Guide: Lose Weight The Healthy Way As Per Ayurveda

Are you sick of pursuing diet after diet without ever reaching your target weight? Perhaps you're just ready for a more holistic approach to weight loss, or you're trying to reset after feeling out of sync with your diet or lifestyle for a short period of time.

Ayurveda offers a straightforward, achievable, and practical approach to weight loss. You'll also be regaining a vibrant feeling of health and well-being along the way. It is always unfailing, consistent, and dependable, as well as incredibly simple to implement.

Ayurvedic weight loss methods may naturally lead us towards holistic and healthy living with no artificial or processed foods or fad diets that damage us more than they help.

A considerable quantity of evidence supports these practices and their significance for weight loss and healthy living. Living an Ayurvedic lifestyle will improve your health and make you more conscious of what you eat, how you move, and how you feel.

This Ayurvedic Weight Loss Guide Covers:
✓Introduction to Ayurveda
✓Reasons for Losing Weight Other than Cosmetic Purposes
✓Common Issues with Diets
✓Ayurveda on Weight Loss
✓Key to Ayurveda's Weight Loss Success
✓Ayurvedic Weight Loss Practices
✓The Role of Routine for Weight Loss

✓Herbs to Boost Your Progress
✓Common Myths and FAQs

So, if you're willing to give an entirely different approach a go, be ready to embark on a new connection with your body as well as an impactful path toward better overall health.

Welcome to the Ayurvedic weight loss approach. This is something you can do. In fact, it may enrich your life in ways that no previous "diet" has ever done.

Slowly but surely, Ayurvedic knowledge will guide you toward stress-free, healthy weight loss.

Reiki For Beginners: The Step-By-Step Guide To Unlock Reiki Self-Healing And Aura Cleansing Secrets For Deep Healing, Peace Of Mind, And Spiritual Growth

Have you always been curious about Reiki? Do you want to witness Reiki in action? Or have you already started your Reiki practice but are looking for additional info? If that's the case, this book is jam-packed with the knowledge that will offer you all you need to know about Reiki so that you may enjoy the benefits of this wonderful practice in your life.

With all the business and technology in our life these days, it is quite simple to have blocked energy. We may be upset about something, neglect our relationships, and do numerous other things. All of this may lead to a variety of physical illnesses and other issues that will not allow us to live healthy or happy life. We may open up our energy and enable it to flow freely through the body using Reiki.

This beginner's guide aims to educate you on how to soothe your mind, body, and soul. You'll be able to ignite your energy and find a strong route to self-attunement and beyond! You will also develop great intuition and clarity, bringing you closer to your inner and spiritual vigor.

This handbook discusses Reiki and how beneficial it may be. Reiki is all around us, and everyone may benefit from its warm, loving energy to help with balance and healing. Because the corpus of information on this topic is so vast, I attempted to condense hundreds of lessons and readings into one easy-to-read book. This book will get you started with Reiki, from the Reiki Symbolism and hand postures through a comprehensive explanation of the various Reiki Techniques.

It will go into how Reiki is an excellent method for moving and healing the energy within our chakras. Reiki practice may cure and reduce pain, both mental and physical, by utilizing vibrations and warmth. You will also have the skills to alter the lives of others if you learn it, and there is nothing more beautiful than compassionate love and healing.

Consider this book to be your insightful Reiki teacher, leading you along your Reiki path to nurture healing. This complete guide includes simple and inclusive training that is comprehensible and accessible to everyone, as well as instructive pictures and guidance that make this book ideal for Reiki students of any age or background.

With this book, you can learn:
✓What Exactly is Reiki?
✓Basics, History, and Principles of Reiki
✓The Energy Centers (Chakras), Their Functioning, and Imbalances
✓The Fundamentals and Knowhow of Kundalini
✓The Meridians in Your Body, How They Interconnect and Affect Us

✓Methods for Resolving Symptoms of Obstructed Energy in Your Mind and Body
✓Reiki's Foundational Pillars
✓The Reiki Advantages
✓Reiki Hand Postures
✓Step-by-Step Reiki Healing
✓Healing Others
✓Reiki Symbols that have the Powerful Healing Forces with Them
✓How Reiki May Significantly Improve Your Health
✓Aura Cleanse and How to Perform An Aura Scan to Feel the Energy in Your Body
✓The Amazing Properties of Crystals and How They Can Boost Your Reiki Practice
✓Tips to Boost Your Reiki Growth
✓Reiki's Most Common FAQs and Myths

Thus, if you are ready to cleanse your energy and experience the happiness and good health that you have been seeking without the use of physicians and medicine, be sure to read this book and learn all you need to get started with Reiki! Don't worry if you're not sure where to begin with spiritual healing. This book will guide you through the recovery process step by step, at your own pace!

More significantly, you will learn how to cleanse your aura and release negativity to promote the universal life force inside your body.

Vipassana Meditation: The Buddhist Mindfulness Practice To Cultivate Joy, Peace, Calmness, And Awakening!!

Are you looking to cultivate true unconditional love towards the creation and experience utter bliss? Do you wish to foster resilience, non-judgment, and detachment? Will you like to master the ancient mindfulness technique that leaded Gautama Buddha to Enlightenment/Nirvana? Do you want to promote relaxation, mindfulness, gratitude, and a better sense of inner peace? Do you want to witness the joy of living in the present moment? If so, Vipassana Meditation is what you need...

Vipassana, which means "seeing things as they really are," is an Indian and Buddhist meditation practice. It was taught over 2500 years ago as a generic cure for universal maladies, i.e., an Art of Living. It is a simple knowledge of what is happening as it is happening.

It is distinct from other forms of meditation practices. The bulk of meditations, whether on a mantra, flame, or activity such as Trataka, are focused on concentration. The practitioner directs his mental energy on an item or a concept. Such methods have validity in terms of relaxing the mind, relaxation, a feeling of well-being, stress reduction, and so on.

Vipassana, in contrast to the other practices, focuses on awareness rather than concentration. Vipassana refers to perceiving reality as it is rather than changing reality, as in concentration practices. The key attribute of Vipassana is its secular nature, which allows it to be practiced by people of any religion, race, caste, nationality, or gender. If the method is to be universal, it must be used by everyone. Here, you concentrate on your breathing, and as you gain control of your breathing observation, you move on to your body responses.

The more the method is used, the more freedom from suffering there is, and the closer one gets to the ultimate objective of complete liberation. Even 10 days may provide effects that are apparent and clearly helpful in daily life.

This step-by-step Vipassana guide takes the reader through

practices that may open new levels of awareness and understanding. This book's aim is to teach you how to live consciously so that you may ultimately be calm and joyful every day of your life!

This is an authentic and practical guide to samatha, materialism, mind, dependent origination, and Vipassana based on the Buddha's teachings. This book will walk you through the stages and methods of overcoming stress, sadness, fear, and anxiety through the practice of Vipassana meditation.

It will explain what this method is and how it came to be. This book also demonstrates how to utilize Vipassana meditation to make our everyday lives more meaningful and, ultimately, to discover the real meaning of peace and tranquillity.

In this book, you'll discover:
✓History of Vipassana Meditation
✓The Deeper Realm of Vipassana
✓The Purpose of Vipassana
✓The Benefits of Vipassana Meditation
✓The Right Attitude Towards the Practice
✓How to Create a Vipassana Retreat at Home
✓The Step-By-Step Vipassana Meditation Practice
✓Tips to Boost Your Progress
✓Additions to Catalyze Your Vipassana Session
✓Beginners Mistakes
✓Common Myths and FAQs
✓Some Pointers from My Experience

Following the instructions in this book will teach you how to develop profound stability, maintain an in-depth study of the intricacies of mind and matter, and ultimately unravel deeply conditioned patterns that perpetuate suffering. It acknowledges with a detailed examination of the different insight and spiritual fruits that the practice offers, Nirvana/Enlightenment being the end goal.

Aromatherapy For Beginners: The Complete Guide To Essential Oils And Aromatherapy To Foster Health, Beauty, Healing, And Well-Being!!

Do you want to fill your home with calming essence and the pleasant smell of nature? Do you wish to get rid of stress and anxiety and relieve various physical and mental conditions? Are you looking to improve your overall physical, mental, emotional, and spiritual health? Do you wish to escalate your spiritual practices? If so, Aromatherapy is what you need...

Even though the word "Aromatherapy" was not coined until the late 1920s, this kind of therapy was found many centuries earlier. The history of the use of essential oils traces back to at least a few thousand years, although human beings have used plants, herbs, etc. for thousands of years. They have been used to improve a person's health or mood for over 6,000 years. Its roots may be traced back to ancient Egypt when fragrant compounds like frankincense and myrrh were utilized in religious and spiritual rituals.

Aromatherapy, often known as essential oil treatment, refers to a group of traditional, alternative, and complementary therapies that make use of essential oils and other aromatic plant components. It is a holistic therapeutic therapy that promotes health and well-being by using natural plant extracts. It employs the therapeutic use of fragrant essential oils to enhance the health of the body, mind, and soul.

Various techniques are used to extract essential or volatile oils from the plant's flowers, bark, stems, leaves, roots, fruits, and other components. It arose as a result of scientists deciphering the antibacterial and skin permeability characteristics of essential oils.

In the modern world, aromatherapy and essential oils have become increasingly popular, not only in the usage of aromatherapy massage and the purchase of pure essential oils but also in the extensive use of essential oils in the cosmetic, skincare, and pharmaceutical industries. Aromatherapy is considered both an art and a science. It provides a variety of medical and psychological advantages, depending on the essential oil or oil combination and manner of application employed.

With this book, I'll share with you every aspect of aromatherapy, as well as the finest techniques you may use to reap the physical, mental, emotional, and spiritual benefits.

This book brings light to the world of aromatherapy by offering a wealth of knowledge and practical guidance on how to get the most out of essential oils. It will offer the best option for living a joyful, natural, healthy, and homeopathic way of life. You will discover a variety of information on the best aromatherapy oils on these pages, including benefits, tips, applications, precautions, myths, and FAQs for using them safely and effectively.

You will discover the science of aromatherapy and how essential oils may totally change your well-being by using the methods mentioned. This book will help you use these potent plant extracts to start feeling better inside and out, no matter where you are on your aromatherapy self-care journey.

In this book, you'll discover:
✓What is Aromatherapy?
✓History and its Significance
✓Aromatherapy Benefits and Conditions it may Treat
✓What are Essential Oils?

✓How are Essential oils Made?
✓The Best Storage Procedure
✓How to Buy Quality Essential Oils?
✓The Best Way to Perform Aromatherapy
✓Activities to perform with Aromatherapy
✓Some Tips that'll Boost Your Progress
✓Essential Oils to Avoid
✓Safety and Precautions
✓Myths and FAQs

So, if you are interested in healing with minimum medication use, spending your time learning about essential oils is a good place to start. Just stick with me until the end to discover how this becomes your ultimate aromatherapy reference and the manifestation of your motives.

The Ayurvedic Dinacharya: Master Your Daily Routine As Per Ayurveda For A Healthy Life And Well-Being!!

Do you wish to synchronize your schedule with nature's rhythm? Do you wish to be disease-free for the rest of your life? Do you want to live a longer, better, and happier life? If yes, this book is going to be an important asset in your life...

Our generation is usually always going through a tough phase. Late nights at work, early meetings, and hectic social life are just a few things that add to our everyday stress. But the main cause for your distress is the lack of a regular schedule. Our forefathers never had to worry about stress since they maintained a disciplined Dinacharya that they followed faithfully. This helps keep the doshas in balance, controls the body's biological cycle, promotes discipline and happiness, and reduces stress.

A lack of routine can also cause many lifestyle disorders such as obesity, hypertension and stroke, diabetes, coronary heart disease, dyslipidemia, cancer, arthritis, anxiety, insomnia, constipation, indigestion, hyperacidity, gastric ulcer, and early manifestations of aging like greying of hair, wrinkles, depletion of energy levels, etc. Simple adjustments in one's lifestyle may prevent these numerous health risks and more.

Dinacharya is formed from two words—'Dina,' which means day, and 'Acharya,' which means activity. By incorporating Dinacharya's basic self-care practices into your life, you will be armed with the skills you need to foster balance, joy, and overall long-term health. It teaches people how to live a better, happier, and longer life while avoiding any illnesses. So irrespective of your body type, age, gender, or health condition, you should opt for a healthy lifestyle.

A daily routine is essential for bringing about a dramatic transformation in the body, mind, and consciousness. Routine aids in the establishment of equilibrium in one's constitution. It also helps with digestion, absorption, and assimilation, as well as generating self-esteem, discipline, tranquility, happiness, and longevity.

With this book, I'll show you how to align yourself with nature's rhythm every day so you may remain healthy and happy for the rest of your life. You will overcome all kinds of mental and physical illnesses in your life. The best part is that these suggestions are centered on Ayurvedic principles and are easy to implement.

This book covers:
✓What is Dinacharya?
✓Importance of Dinacharya
✓Dinacharya Benefits
✓Daily Cycles and Dinacharya
✓The Morning Dinacharya

✓The Afternoon and Sundown Dinacharya
✓The Evening and Night Dinacharya
✓How to Implement Dinacharya into Your Life?
✓Tips to Boost Your Progress
✓Beginners Dinacharya Mistakes

This book is perfect for anybody seeking simple, all-encompassing methods to live a more genuine and balanced life. You'll discover techniques and ideas to help you stay calm, balanced, and joyful.

Shadow Work For Beginners: A Short And Powerful Guide To Make Peace With Your Hidden Dark Side That Drive You And Illuminate The Hidden Power Of Your True Self For Freedom And Lasting Happiness

Do you want to recognize and heal the shadow patterns and wounds of your inner child? Do you wish to get rooted in your soul for wholeness? Do you want to influence your programs and beliefs to attain eternal bliss? Do you want to know where you are on the ladder of consciousness, and how to move up? Do you want to learn how to forgive, let go, and have compassion for yourself and others? Do you want to alter and strengthen your mindset to maximize every aspect of your life? If so, this guide is just what you need.

For many, the word "shadow work" conjures up all sorts of negative and dark ideas. Because of the beliefs we have of the term shadow, it is tempting to believe that shadow work is a morbid spiritual practice or that it is an internal work that includes the more destructive or evil facets of our personalities. But that's not the case. In fact, shadow work is vital to your spiritual growth. When you go through a spiritual awakening, there comes a point where "shadow work" becomes necessary.

So, what exactly is the 'Human Shadow,' and what is 'Shadow Work?'

The definition of the shadow self is based on the idea that we figuratively bury certain bits of personality that we feel will not be embraced, approved, or cherished by others; thus, we hold them in the "shadows." In brief, our shadows are the versions of ourselves that we do not offer society.

It includes aspects of our personality that we find shameful, unacceptable, ugly. It may be anger, resentment, frustration, greed, hunger for strength, or the wounds of childhood—all those we hold secret. You might claim it's the dark side of yourself. And no matter what everyone suggests, they all have a dark side of their personalities.

Shadow Work is the practice of loving what is, and of freeing shame and judgment, so that we can be our true self in order to touch the very depths of our being, that is what Shadow Work means. You have to dwell on the actual problems rather than on past emotions. If you do so, you get to the problems that have you stressed out instantly and easily. And to be at peace, we need to get in touch with our darker side, rather than suppressing it.

Whether you have struggled with wealth, weight, love, or something else, after dissolving the shadows within, you will find that your life is transforming in both tiny and drastic ways. You'll draw more optimistic people and better opportunities. Your life will be nicer, easier, and even more abundant.

The book covers the easiest practices and guided meditation to tap into the unconscious. It's going to help you explore certain aspects so that they will no longer control your emotions. Just imagine what it would be if you could see challenges as exciting obstacles rather than experiencing crippling anxiety.

This book is going to be the Momentum you need to get to where you're trying to be. You'll go deeper into your thoughts, the beliefs that hold you back disappear, and you get a head start on your healing journey.

In this guide, you'll discover:

✓What is the Human Shadow?
✓Characteristics of Shadow
✓Do We All Have a Shadow Self?
✓How is The Shadow Born?
✓What is the Golden Shadow?
✓The Mistake We All Make
✓What is Shadow Work?
✓Benefits of Shadow Work
✓Tips on Practicing Shadow Work
✓Shadow Work Stages
✓Shadow Work Techniques and Practices
✓Shadow Work Mindfulness
✓Shadow Work FAQs

Covering every bit of Shadow Work, this guide will subtly reveal the root of your fear, discomfort, and suffering, showing you that when you allow certain pieces of yourself to awaken and be, you will eventually begin to recover, transcend your limits, and open yourself to the light and beauty of your true existence.

Spiritual Empath: The Ultimate Guide To Awake Your Maximum Capacity And Have That Power, Compassion, And Wisdom Contained In Your Soul

Do you keep attracting toxic individuals and set a poor barrier? Do you get consumed by negative emotions and feel like you can't deal with it? Do you want to heal yourself and seek inner peace and spiritual growth? If so, this book is going to open the doors for you!!

Empaths have too much to contribute as healers, creators, friends, lovers, and innovators at work. Yet extremely compassionate and empathic people sometimes give too much at the cost of their own well-being-and end up consuming the stress of others. Why?

These questions and more will be addressed in this book. You'll find the answers you're searching for to learn the facts on whether you're an empath, how it can work on a biological level, what to do to help you succeed as an empath, and how to shield yourself from other people's thoughts, feelings, and responses so that you don't absorb them.

There is a lot of things going in the life of empaths, and they are here to add more happiness and peace to the world. Empaths are known for their willingness to listen, sensitivity, empathy, and the capacity to be in the shoes of others. You may be that individual, or you might know that individual in your life, but either way, knowing the true cause of being an empath and why they are different from others will help you improve to lead a healthy, free, and beautiful life full of empathy.

This book includes the following, and much more:

✓What is an Empath?
✓Are You an Empath?
✓Is Being an Empath a Gift or Disorder
✓The List of Empath Superpowers
✓Ways to Turn Your Super Traits into Super Powers
✓The Secret Dark Side of Being an Empath
✓What It's Like Being an Intuitive/Psychic Empath
✓Signs You're the Most Powerful Empath (Heyoka)
✓Is Your Soul Exhausted and Energy Depleted?
✓Tips To Become an Empath Warrior

✓Empath's Survival Guide/Tips to Stay Balanced as an Empath
✓Ways to Save Yourself from Narcissists
✓Best Practices to Deal with Anxiety
✓Why Self-Love/Self-Care is So Important
✓Empath Awakening Stages
✓Best Transmutation Techniques for Raising Your Energies and Vibrations for Spiritual Growth

Right now, you can opt to proceed on a profound healing path and find strength in the deep pockets of your soul. Or you might want to put off the re-discovery of your inner voice and intuition, feeling like you might never have had it; never really understood how your powerful empathic ability can be channeled for the greatest benefit of all, including your own highest gain.

Filled with lots of insight into the inner workings of Empath's mind, useful knowledge to help you make sense of your abilities, and keep negative individuals and energies out of your life. This book contains all you need to become a stronger, better version of yourself.

That's correct, with this book, you can move out of your usual role and begin a journey. You'll experience the emergence of the inner energies and become a spiritually awakened person.

Meditation For Beginners: The Easiest Guide To Cultivate Awareness, Acceptance, And Peace To Unleash Your Inner Strength And Explore The Deepest Realm Of Your Being!!

Whether you're looking to increase self-awareness, reduce negative emotions, bust stress, promote creativity, foster good health and mental peace, or transcend the limitations of human life and connect with universal forces to see the transcendental reality through it (called Brahman in the Vedas), meditation solves all…

It is estimated that 200–500 million individuals meditate across the globe. Meditation statistics suggest that the practice has grown in popularity in recent years. Given all the health advantages it provides, it's no wonder that a rising number of individuals are using it. Through it, more and more people are recognizing a profound inner longing for authenticity, connection, compassion, and aliveness.

Meditation may seem to be a simple concept—sit still, focus on your breath, and observe. However, the practice of meditation has a long cultural history that has seen it evolve from a religious concept to something that might today seem more alluring than spiritual. It is a centuries-old technique that is said to have started in India thousands of years ago. Throughout history, the practice was gradually adopted by neighboring nations and became a part of numerous religions around the globe.

The goal of meditation is to become consciously aware of or explore one's own mind and body to get to know oneself. It is fundamentally both an exclusive and inclusive process in which one withdraws one's thoughts and senses from the distractions of the world and concentrates on a selected object or idea.

It is focused attention, with or without an individual's will, in which the mind and body must be brought together to work as one harmonic whole. We may overcome mental obstacles, negative thinking, crippling worries, tension, and anxiety with the aid of meditation by understanding and dealing with the underlying causes. We gain insightful awareness in meditation, allowing us to manage our responses and reactions.

So, whether you want to ease stress, attain spiritual

enlightenment, seek peace, or flow through movement, meditation is the way to go.

But how will we know which meditation practice is best for us as there are plenty of them?? While there are various types of meditation, each takes you to the same spot. It's like there are various routes to the same destination. So, it didn't matter which route you take. Here in this book, I'll discuss a certain type of meditation that I found to be the easiest and most effective.

Although there is no right or incorrect method to meditate, it is important to select a practice that matches your requirements and compliments your nature. And the type of meditation I'm going to discuss here is ideal for anyone—from beginners to advanced.

The practice will inject far-reaching and long-lasting advantages into your life—lower stress, more awareness of your struggles, better ability to connect, enhanced awareness, and being nicer to yourself are just some of its benefits.

In this book, you'll discover:
✓What is Meditation?
✓Meditation Benefits
✓The Role of Diet in Meditation
✓Various Mudras
✓Various Asanas
✓The Ideal Setting for Meditation
✓How Yoga and Pranayamas can Help Boost the Practice?
✓The Easiest Meditation Practice
✓The Wrong Way to Approach Meditation
✓The Right Way to Approach Meditation
✓The Significance of Keeping the Spine Straight
✓The Importance of Breath Rhythm
✓Some Tips to Enhance the Practice
✓How Group Meditation is Better than Meditating Alone?

✓The Significance of Routine
✓How to Bring Meditation to Daily Life Activities?
✓Common Meditation Myths and FAQs
✓Some Tips from Experience

So, if you're ready, claim your copy right now and embark on this quest beyond yourself...

Who Are You: The Spiritual Awakening Self Discovery Guide For Enlightenment And Liberation (Available For Free!!)

Have you ever thought after reaching your goal, why aren't you happy? It's because that is not what you need to be happy.

The major problem today in this world is that everyone is searching for joy in materialistic objects like money, fame, respect, and whatever. But the fact is, the most successful personalities in the world which you admire so much are not happy at all! If that was the case, they won't ever get depressed or sad. Is that what the reality is? No, in fact, they're the one who takes depression therapies and drugs to be happy.

What are all the fundamental problems that we all face? There is a sense of lack that exists in all of us, a sense of loneliness, a sense of incompleteness, a sense of being restricted, a sense of fear, fear of death. So these fundamental problems can only be overcome through self-investigation; there's no other way around.

Being happy is a basic nature of human beings, just like the basic nature of fire is hot. But the error we make is we're searching for happiness outside, which is impossible to achieve. Say, you wanted something for a very long time; what happens after you achieve it? You'll be happy for a while, but then you'll need something else to be happy, you'll then run after some other goal; it's an endless cycle!

The good thing is, there's a way to be happy at every moment, but to make it happen you must understand in a peaceful state of mind "Who Are You?"
You'll have to self-enquire! This book is based on one of the most popular Indian Scripture "Ashtavakra Geeta" that reveals the ultimate truth of mankind. It will open the doors for you on how we can achieve self-knowledge and be fearless. All your fears and doubts will come to an end; not temporarily, but forever. All internal conflicts will fall to zero, and psychological pain will cease to exist.

This is not just another self-help book; this spiritual workbook will help you achieve liberation and be self-enlightened!

Reading this book:
✓You'll attain everlasting peace
✓You'll understand the real meaning of spiritual awakening
✓You'll understand spirituality over religion
✓You'll get the answer to 'Who Are You?'
✓You'll be fearless
✓You'll be free from bondage and be able to achieve liberation
✓You'll get the key to everlasting happiness and joy
✓You'll grasp the real essence of spirituality and the awakening self
✓You'll get to know about spirituality for the skeptic
✓You'll discover your higher self
✓You'll be able to experience the joy of self-realization
✓You'll find what spiritual enlightenment means in Buddhism
✓You'll know how to achieve or reach spiritual enlightenment
✓You'll know what happens after spiritual enlightenment
✓You'll get the answer to why you should have spiritual awakening

And this is a book not just for adults but also for kids and teens.

Chakras For Beginners: A Guide To Understanding 7 Chakras Of The Body: Nourish, Heal, And Fuel The Chakras For Higher Consciousness And Awakening! (Available For Free!!)

Chakras are the circular vortexes of energy that are placed in seven different points on the spinal column, and all the seven chakras are connected to the various organs and glands within the body. These chakras are responsible for disturbing the life energy, which is also known as Qi or Praana.

Chakras have more than one dimension to them. One dimension is their physical existence, but they also have a spiritual dimension. Whenever a chakra is disrupted or blocked, the life energy also gets blocked, leading to the onset of mental and health ailments. When the harmonious balance of the seven chakras is disrupted or damaged, it can cause several problems in our lives, including our physical health, emotional health, and our mental state of mind. If all our chakras are balanced and in harmony, our body will function in an optimum way; If unbalanced, our energies will be like in a small river where the water will flow irregularly and noisily. By balancing our chakras, the water/our energies will flow more freely throughout our bodies and thus the risk of imbalances and consequent illnesses will be reduced to a minimum.

In this book, I'm going to give you an excellent resource you can use to amplify the work you do with your chakras.

In this book you'll learn:

✓The Number of Chakras in Our Body (Not 7)

✓The Location of Chakras
✓Meaning Related to Each Chakra
✓Color Psychology
✓How to Balance the Chakras
✓Characteristics/Impacts of Each Chakra When Balanced and Imbalanced
✓Aspects of Nature
✓Qualities
✓Gemstones to Support Each Chakra

Step-By-Step Beginners Instant Pot Cookbook (Vegan): 100+ Easy, Delicious Yet Extremely Healthy Instant Pot Recipes Backed By Ayurveda Which Anyone Can Make In Less Than 30 Minutes

Who said healthy foods can't be tasty, I am a health-conscious person and love to eat healthy food, as well as tasty food.

"You Don't Have to Cook Fancy or Complicated Masterpieces. Just Tasty Food From Simple Healthy Ingredients."

Well, you don't have to struggle anymore with the taste. Here in this cookbook, you'll find 100+ easy yet extremely delicious instant pot recipes. keeping in mind the health factor, all these recipes are backed by Ayurveda, so yes, all are highly nutritious as well.

If you follow Ayurveda you know why we shouldn't eat meat or non-veg, so finally here is a Complete Vegan Instant Pot Cookbook. Plus, these do not require ingredients that'll hurt your budget, nearly all the ingredients are readily available in your home.

Every recipe is properly portioned and will be ready in 30 minutes or less. These quick and simple recipes will get your meal ready on the table in no time.

In this Instant Pot Cookbook you will find:

✓ Insider's Knowledge on How to Make the Most Out of Your Instant Pot
✓ Common FAQs and Other Must-Know Facts about Your Instant Pot
✓ Pro Tips to Get the Most out of Your Instant pot
✓ Things Not to Do with Your Instant Pot
✓ No Non-Veg, Complete Vegan Recipes
✓ How to Create a Variety of Healthy, Easy-to-Make, Delicious Recipes in the Easiest Way Possible

No matter if you're a solo eater, or if you cook for the whole family or friends, with these easy and healthy recipes, you can surprise your family, friends, and your loved ones.

This cookbook includes delicious recipes for:

✓Breakfast Meals
✓Stews and Chilies
✓Soups
✓Beans
✓Lunch/Brunch
✓Side Meals
✓Main Course Meals
✓Appetizers & Snacks
✓Light Dinner
✓Deserts
✓Bonus Recipes Including Salads, Drinks, and Some of the Most Popular Indian Dishes